# CREATIVE WAYS TO HELP
# CHILDREN MANAGE ANXIETY

# CREATIVE WAYS
## TO HELP CHILDREN MANAGE ANXIETY

IDEAS AND ACTIVITIES FOR WORKING
THERAPEUTICALLY WITH WORRIED
CHILDREN AND THEIR FAMILIES

**DR. FIONA ZANDT AND DR. SUZANNE BARRETT**

FOREWORD BY DR. KAREN CASSIDAY
ILLUSTRATIONS BY RICHY K. CHANDLER

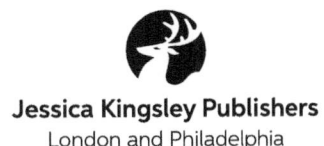

**Jessica Kingsley Publishers**
London and Philadelphia

First published in Great Britain in 2021 by Jessica Kingsley Publishers

An Hachette Company

1

A CIP catalogue record for this title is available from the British Library and the Library of Congress

ISBN 978 1 78775 094 4
eISBN 978 1 78775 095 1

Printed and bound in the Great Britain by TJ International Ltd

Jessica Kingsley Publishers' policy is to use papers that are natural, renewable and recyclable
products and made from wood grown in sustainable forests. The logging and manufacturing
processes are expected to conform to the environmental regulations of the country of origin.

Jessica Kingsley Publishers
73 Collier Street
London N1 9BE, UK

www.jkp.com

*To Megan, Harry and Larni—with all my love. And to James, Joseph, Christian and Edith – as always.*

FZ


*To Mum and Dad, and to Arch, Alyssa, Annabelle and Bradley—with love and thanks for all of your support.*

SB

# Contents

# Therapeutic Activities

# Acknowledgements

We are incredibly grateful to all of the children and families we have had the privilege to work with. Thank you for continuing to challenge us to remain playful and creative in all we do.

We are also thankful to have worked alongside and learnt so much from our many wonderful colleagues over the years. In particular we wish to thank Associate Professor Lesley Bretherton and Dr. Maree Dellaportas for their helpful feedback on this book.

Our sincere thanks to Jane Evans, our editor, for her support and guidance. We'd also like to thank the rest of the Jessica Kingsley Publishers team, including Simeon Hance, Karina Maduro and Pippa Adams, for all their help in producing and supporting the ongoing distribution of our books. Thank you for enabling us to share our learning with therapists across the globe and in doing so, to help more children and families.

Most of all, we are grateful to our families—without their love and support none of this would have been possible.

# Foreword

One of the most difficult challenges for any child and adolescent therapist who works with anxious children is trying to make appealing a fundamentally unappealing task. The task of teaching children and their parents to face and manage their anxiety goes against the child's instinct to avoid and the parent's desire to comfort. Evidence-based interventions for children necessitate therapeutic exposure to the very feelings and situations that the child, and even their parents, believes to be impossible. Having strategies that offer the possibilities for fun and that harness a child's imagination and spirit of learning through play have a great advantage over simply offering rewards for participation in treatment. Children, and quite frankly adults, all learn better by doing. Children also naturally use play to explore things that are challenging, difficult to understand and distressing. That means that any therapist who works with children is going to have to figure out how to incorporate play, good humor and imagination to help children acquire the skills to overcome anxiety successfully.

The other dilemma that many therapists face is that they have spent a lot of time in school, including graduate school. This means that they have likely had the fun beaten out of them and have spent many hours engaged in a type of learning that emphasizes listening to an expert pontificate, focussing upon gaining a new graduate level of vocabulary, known as professional jargon, and being very serious. Therapists have also probably spent very little time playing, watching kid-related media and doing the things that make it easy to be spontaneous, silly and, quite frankly, kid-attractive. It is also likely that their graduate training emphasized following a particular protocol that did not focus upon play but instead focussed upon treatment fidelity. They may have been told to offer candy or stickers at the end of every session, but this is often a poor motivation for a child who is freaking out with panic and can only imagine how to flee your office. Sadly, these are not the skills that make clinicians kid-friendly.

So, if you want to succeed with kids, then you are going to have to learn how to play, to dance, to sing, to be silly and to speak without using jargon. You are going to have to forget about giving brilliant explanations and remember that kids learn best when they discover what works, when they use their imagination and when they view therapy as an adventure. Play is what makes this possible.

I invite you to enjoy this wonderful book that Dr. Zandt and Dr. Barrett have created for all of us grownup therapists who need a kickstart for our imagination. Dr. Zandt and

Dr. Barrett have taken the complicated ideas that explain how anxiety works in the body and mind and created fun, memorable ways to explain and experience what happens when a child gets anxious and what to do once anxiety occurs. I love being playful and using play with my young patients because it puts the emphasis on joyful exploration and learning and takes the child's attention away from waiting for the next painful moment. We can all improve our therapist play skills, because our status as grownups who must constantly learn at a graduate level compromises our ability to be playful. This book is one that I am sure you will enjoy as you implement its suggestions with your patients and both discover how joyful it is to overcome anxiety, kid-style!

*Dr. Karen Cassiday*

# Preface

Worries and fears are a normal part of childhood. However, at times anxiety reaches a point where it becomes problematic for children. Anxiety disorders are the most common mental health conditions affecting children, are often chronic and are associated with mental health difficulties in adulthood (Farrell, Ollendick and Muris 2019).

Anxiety, in its many forms, is one of the most common reasons that children and families present for therapy. Untreated it can have a significant impact on many areas of a child's development and can result in marked stress and strain for families. As therapists we need to be able to work well with children with anxiety and their families. In this book we outline our playful, purposeful and practical ideas for working therapeutically with children with anxiety.

First, and perhaps most essentially, our approach with children is playful. Play is a child's natural form of communication. It provides them with many essential skills, including learning about relationships, developing self-regulation, learning to negotiate and repair, assessing risk, making sense of their world and practicing new behaviors or roles. Piaget (2000) contended that children learn best when they are actively involved, doing and exploring, and using play in therapy is a great way to help children learn about therapeutic concepts. In therapy we scaffold for the child, supporting their learning and allowing them to engage more with therapeutic concepts than they are able to do independently. We create what Vygotsky (1986) referred to as the zone of proximal development, in which a child can learn through interacting with someone who is more experienced. Play also provides opportunities for practice and repetition, while encouraging flexibility. For example, a child who is engaged in a role play can try out different ways of responding to worries.

Perhaps most importantly, play is engaging, calming and fun for children. This aspect of play should not be underestimated. Having fun in therapy ensures that children feel helpful about coming and makes it more likely that they will want to come again. For some children the opportunity to share enjoyable time with a supportive and caring adult will be a rare experience, and in some instances this may be the most valuable contribution of our therapy time with the child.

Being playful requires us to be open and flexible, to not be focussed on competence, and instead be immersed in the process. One aspect of being playful is that we share a little of ourselves in the play. For example, when talking about the child's feelings, we would share a little about our own feelings, taking care to share only what is appropriate and supports the child's therapy. Some therapists are naturally more playful than others and sometimes this is understandable in the context of our own play history. The same will also be true for the parents we work with. Noticing your own tendencies and finding ways to work that suit your style and setting is important.

We use play in a directed way to help children understand and explore therapeutic concepts. We use a cognitive behavioral therapy (CBT) approach (including acceptance and commitment therapy) with systemic family therapy and narrative therapy influences. Our approach is therefore purposeful. We remain goal-focussed, being clear about the therapeutic concepts we want to work on with children. The goals are derived from our understanding of the child and their difficulties with anxiety in the context of their family and broader systems. As therapists we often think of this as our formulation; and regardless of the model we are trained in, this emphasizes the importance of assessment. Completing a comprehensive assessment and sharing our understanding with the family provides a space in which we can develop goals and keep our therapy focussed and purposeful.

A final aspect of our approach is that we work in a way that is practical. A practical approach recognizes how busy life is for children and families, providing strategies that fit within this. For example, it is not useful to suggest that a child use some sensory calming strategies at preschool if the teacher is not supportive of this. Similarly, it is unlikely to be effective for a busy family to do a 15-minute relaxation exercise daily; however, it might be practical for them to model a single deep breath and pause in difficult situations. We work closely with families throughout therapy, and when we refer to families we are referring to whoever the child lives with. When we talk about parents in this book we are talking about whoever is in the caregiving role.

Keeping therapy practical increases the likelihood that children and families will stay engaged. This is particularly true for parents who are often very concerned and stressed by the time they come to therapy. Having something useful and manageable that they can do is often containing for parents and supports them to engage with the therapy process. Some children too can be unsure about the point of therapy and feel frustrated about missing out on school or other activities. Keeping therapy practical and focussed is often important in keeping these children engaged.

Making therapy practical for therapists is also an important consideration. Therapy ideas that require extensive preparation, are costly or use difficult to source materials are less likely to be implemented by therapists. In addition, many therapists work in a mobile context, visiting children at school or at home, meaning that they need activities that include few materials, which are easily transportable. We also use materials in more than one context, meaning that traveling therapists can pack up a minimal number of materials and utilize these for numerous activities.

More generally, many therapists work in contexts in which our involvement with clients is short term due to funding or organizational constraints. Being able to make a difference within a short amount of time matters, so keeping our approach practical and focussed is often useful. We are also mindful that mental health difficulties, and indeed the need for intervention, can disrupt a child's development. Keeping therapy practical and focussed tends to mean we can have the greatest impact in the least amount of time, allowing children to return to doing the things we want them to be doing—regular things like attending school, playing with their brothers and sisters, hanging out with friends and playing sports.

This book provides background information on childhood anxiety and ideas for working with anxious children, aged 4–12 years, in a playful, purposeful and practical manner. Hypothetical case descriptions are included throughout to illustrate this. Fiona is the primary author and first-person references throughout the text refer to her practice and experience. Key interventions for helping children with anxiety are presented, along with 55 creative therapeutic activities which are written up with ideas about how to present these to children and how to involve families.

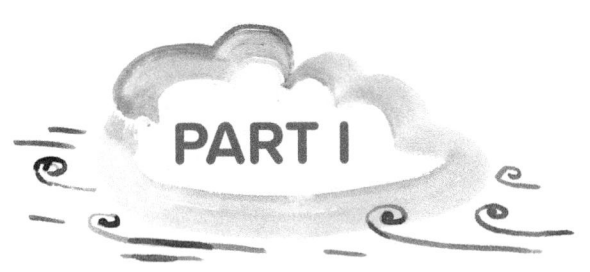

PART I

# A PLAYFUL, PURPOSEFUL AND PRACTICAL APPROACH TO CHILDHOOD ANXIETY

# CHAPTER 1

# ANXIETY IN CHILDREN

### RIVER

River was a 10-year-old boy who presented with generalized worries, a fear of vomiting and anxiety about performance situations. He was a well-liked and academically competent boy who avoided performance situations at school—for example, speaking in front of his class. His anxiety about being judged negatively by his peers and teacher meant that he missed out on the learning and development that would come from sharing his ideas with others. His fear of making a mistake further prevented him from having a go and trying out ideas. Although he loved football, he became reluctant to play matches with his team, as he was anxious about being watched and having his skills judged negatively. He eventually withdrew from football, missing further opportunities to build confidence, physical skills and friendships, and to have fun through his sport.

All children experience anxiety or worry from time to time. Indeed, some anxiety is helpful, having an essential role in alerting us and protecting us from danger. For example, having some anxiety about strangers keeps us safe. Anxiety can have a function, provided it isn't excessive and doesn't cause us distress or get in the way of what we want or need to do. For example, a child who has a small amount of worry about an upcoming spelling test is likely to practice their words and will probably focus well on the day of the test.

Anxiety is common in children. A meta-analysis of 41 studies across 27 countries found the worldwide-pooled prevalence of anxiety disorders in children and adolescents to be 6.5%, with anxiety disorders being the most common group of mental disorders in young people (Polanczyk *et al.* 2015). This is consistent with a recent US estimate suggesting that 7.1% of children aged 3–17 years had a current anxiety disorder (Ghandour *et al.* 2019). It is also consistent with the Young Minds Matter Survey, a recent, national Australian survey that found 6.6% of 4–17-year-olds had a separation anxiety, social anxiety or generalized anxiety disorder (Spence, Zubrick and Lawrence 2018). In their international review, Polanczyk *et al.* (2015) found that prevalence estimates varied related to sample characteristics and how the studies assessed anxiety, though not according to the location or year of the studies. Anxiety is clearly a common challenge for many children and is one that child therapists are frequently engaged in treating.

Anxiety has a ripple effect and can impact on many other areas of a child's life. A child who is missing school as a result of separation anxiety is likely to miss out on lots of social interaction, learning and the opportunity for independence, meaning that the impact is far-reaching. If the child does not attend school for a long time, social and academic difficulties can result. Similarly, a child who is fearful of making mistakes may avoid tasks they perceive as difficult and as a result not only will their learning suffer but they also won't discover that they can be anxious and do something anyway. In the longer term, anxiety impacts on the way in which a child sees both the world and themselves. It shapes the way that the family perceive a child too, often impacting on how they relate.

Cognitive, emotional and social development is constantly shaping the way in which a child perceives their world. This means that children are more likely to develop different kinds of anxiety at different stages. For example, separation anxiety tends to be most apparent early in life when children first begin to spend time away from their families. As imagination develops in preschool-aged children, worries about monsters, witches and the dark become pronounced. Fears of physical injury, animals and storms are common, and children's awareness of the finality of death may also emerge. In the primary school years, as children become more aware of current affairs, we see more general worries. Children in this age group might worry about illness, disasters, or the death of or harm to a parent, and worries related to school and performance may emerge. Social development in adolescence involves an increased focus on peer acceptance, which can be associated with the onset of social anxiety. Table 1.1 outlines some of the normative fears we see in each age group as well as common diagnoses for anxiety that has become problematic.

Table 1.1 Development, normal fears and anxiety disorders

| Age | Normative fears | Common diagnoses |
|---|---|---|
| Infancy and toddlerhood (under 3 years) | Separation<br>Strangers | |
| Preschool age (3–6 years) | Thunder and lightning<br>Fire or water<br>Darkness or nightmares<br>Imaginary creatures<br>Animals<br>Dying or death of others | Specific phobias<br>Separation anxiety disorder<br>Selective mutism |
| School age (6–12 years) | Germs and illness<br>Natural disasters<br>Traumatic events<br>Harm to self or others<br>School anxiety<br>Performance anxiety | Generalized anxiety disorder<br>Obsessive compulsive disorder |
| Adolescence (over 12 years) | Fear of negative evaluation<br>Rejection from peers | Social anxiety disorder<br>Panic disorder |

*Adapted from Carr (2016) and Beesdo-Baum and Knappe (2012).*

The *Diagnostic and Statistical Manual of Mental Disorders 5th edition* (*DSM-5*; American Psychiatric Association 2013) and the *International Statistical Classification of Diseases and Related Health Problems 11th edition* (*ICD-11*; World Health Organization 2019) list a number of anxiety disorders, including separation anxiety disorder and selective mutism, which typically occur in children. The other anxiety disorders listed—specific phobias, social anxiety disorder, generalized anxiety disorder, panic disorder and agoraphobia— can also be diagnosed in childhood. A number of other disorders included in the *DSM-5* and *ICD-11* are worth noting here too, as anxiety remains a central component of their presentation. These include posttraumatic stress disorder (PTSD) and obsessive compulsive disorder (OCD). The box below provides a brief description of these disorders.

## Anxiety Disorders

**SEPARATION ANXIETY DISORDER**
Excessive anxiety concerning separation from those individuals to whom the child is attached.

**SELECTIVE MUTISM**
Consistent failure to speak in specific social situations in which there is an expectation for speaking (e.g., at preschool) despite speaking in other situations (e.g., at home).

**SPECIFIC PHOBIA**
Marked fear or anxiety about a specific object or situation (e.g., heights, blood or a particular animal).

**SOCIAL ANXIETY DISORDER**
Marked fear or anxiety about social situations in which the child is exposed to possible scrutiny by peers.

**GENERALIZED ANXIETY DISORDER**
Excessive worry about a number of events or activities (e.g., school performance) with associated anxiety symptoms.

**PANIC DISORDER**
Unexpected panic attacks, and either worry about additional panic attacks or changes in behavior related to the attacks.

**AGORAPHOBIA**
Marked fear or anxiety about at least two of the following situations (where it is difficult to escape or find help if experiencing symptoms): public transport, open spaces, enclosed places, being in crowds or lines, or outside of the home alone.

**OBSESSIVE COMPULSIVE DISORDER (OCD)**

Presence of obsessions, compulsions, or both. Obsessions are recurrent and persistent thoughts, urges or images that are experienced as intrusive and unwanted. Compulsions are repetitive behaviors or mental acts performed in response to an obsession or according to rigid rules.

**POSTTRAUMATIC STRESS DISORDER (PTSD)**

Exposure to actual or threatened death, serious injury or sexual violence (excluding through media) with associated symptoms of intrusion, avoidance and negative alterations in cognitions, mood, arousal and reactivity.

**COMPLEX POSTTRAUMATIC STRESS DISORDER (COMPLEX PTSD; *ICD-11* ONLY)**

Exposure to an event or series of events of an extremely threatening or horrific nature, which are commonly prolonged or repetitive. In addition to PTSD symptoms, complex PTSD is characterized by severe and persistent symptoms related to affect regulation, relationships, self-beliefs and shame, guilt or failure.

(Adapted from *DSM-5*, American Psychiatric Association 2013; and *ICD-11*, World Health Organization 2019)

Increasingly, developmental trauma is being written about. Many children will experience anxiety, having been raised in environments that are unpredictable, chaotic and frightening. For these children much of their anxiety occurs at a non-verbal level, having been experienced prior to an age and stage when they were verbal. Some of these children might fit the criteria for complex PTSD, introduced in *ICD-11*, or an attachment disorder (reactive attachment disorder or disinhibited social engagement disorder), though some may not. Ensuring that children are safe and well supported is essential for those who have experienced developmental trauma. Provided some of this initial work has been undertaken and the therapist remains mindful of the child's early experiences throughout therapy, many of the activities in this book can be adapted for use in this context. Indeed, the nature of trauma is such that supporting a child to better understand and manage their anxiety is often an essential aspect of therapy. Driggs McLeod (2018) explains that "targeting anxiety advances and informs an array of other goals that promote a restoration of improved general functioning postabuse" (p.244). Often when children have experienced trauma there are ongoing stressors they are likely to be faced with. For example, a child who has been removed from her parents as a result of abuse is likely to experience anxiety about her wellbeing and that of her parents, anxiety about her new carers, and anxiety around visitation and other processes associated with the separation. In the longer term she is likely to face additional challenges and stressors. Helping children to develop coping strategies is essential in this context, as is building supportive relationships between children and their carers. Hence, most of what we discuss is relevant for children who have experienced trauma.

## Core features of anxiety

### JOHN

John was a 5-year-old boy who was referred for controlling behavior and angry outbursts. Upon assessment, however, it was clear that his controlling behavior centered on him insisting that his parents stay in the same room with him at home and sleep with him at night, and his angry outbursts occurred in the mornings prior to him attending school. In therapy John was able to articulate some of his worries about being away from his parents, which changed the way in which they understood his behavior and allowed them to engage in interventions around his anxiety.

Anxiety has some core components that are apparent regardless of the diagnosis. This includes affective responses, physiological reactions, cognitive processes and behavioral responses. We will discuss each of these in turn.

## Affective responses

Many children who are anxious describe being worried or scared. However, at times other feelings may be expressed. Anxiety is often felt as a sense of dread, or a persistent feeling of nervousness, which may be displayed as uneasiness or irritability. Sometimes in children who have experienced trauma, we see emotional blunting, where they seem to display little emotion and instead feel numb, perhaps while experiencing episodes of intense emotions at other times. Some children, especially those who are younger, may not be able to verbalize their emotions, though we may observe their distress and discomfort.

As in the example above, anxiety can also be expressed as anger and this is a reaction that we often observe in children. Often it appears to be a way for the child to release their feelings and frequently the anger is channeled toward other areas rather than the focus of the worry. For example, a child who is worried about a presentation at school may become angry about little things, such as not having his favorite breakfast cereal or his mother not buttering his toast properly. Helping parents to identify these patterns and tune into the underlying anxiety is important.

## Physiological responses

### KATIE

Katie was a 12-year-old girl with separation anxiety and generalized anxiety who had previously been unable to engage in therapy. She had responded well to medication, with her symptoms decreasing by the time the family attempted therapy again. Despite this, Katie found talking about her feelings and thoughts difficult. She would yawn frequently and felt very tired during the sessions. It seemed that Katie was experiencing a fatigue response to her anxiety in the sessions. The therapist was able to reflect on her difficulty talking about her experience and wonder about how this related to what was happening in her body. Katie became increasingly able to talk about this, and she and the therapist had playful interactions around noticing the first time she would yawn each session.

A flight, fight or freeze response represents the physiological component of anxiety, which has evolutionary value in preparing our body for danger. A flight response would involve running away from your predator, whereas a fight response would involve preparing to physically fight for your survival. A freeze response involves an attempt to protect yourself by playing dead and disconnecting from the dangerous reality. These responses in our body are triggered when we feel anxious. The flight or fight response activates and powers our body, increasing our breathing and heart rate to send blood and oxygen to our muscles to prepare us for fighting or running. The freeze response in contrast lowers heart rate and blood pressure as a protective function and can sometimes induce a dissociative state. A simple, child-friendly explanation of the fight or flight response and its protective function can be found in the picture book *Hey Warrior* by Karen Young, illustrated by Norvile Dovidonyte (2016). The freeze response is also important to consider, particularly for those children with developmental trauma. Treisman (2016) covers this topic in depth for the interested reader.

Often we see children having similar patterns. For example, although a flight response is typically thought of as running away, many children may simply refuse to participate in a task. A child who refuses to go on the ride or attempt a project is displaying a flight or avoidance pattern. Some children will also engage in fight responses, though these are not always physical. For example, a child who is anxious about going onstage might verbally fight over their costume not being right or how their hair has been done. Finally, some children will freeze when anxious, a bit like a rabbit caught in headlights. This response can be particularly true of children who have experienced trauma. A related response is fatigue, which may be experienced as an overwhelming desire for a nap, as we saw Katie experience in the example above.

The flight or fight response means that we often see anxious children with a heightened level of arousal in their bodies. They may seem agitated and find it difficult to stay still, or they may jump in response to being startled, hold a lot of tension in their muscles, or be constantly looking all around. They may appear "on edge" and can be described as hypervigilant. Some children are constantly on the lookout for danger, which can prevent them from enjoying interactions and activities. We observe this pattern in anxious children, and particularly those whose anxiety occurs in the context of trauma, who have not had the experience of feeling safe in their environment. Those who are interested in learning more about the impact of trauma on children might like to read Perry and Szalavitz (2017) and Treisman (2016).

The hyperarousal that anxious children experience can lead to somatic complaints such as chest pain, muscle tension, headaches, stomachaches and nausea (Rapee 2012; Stallard 2009). These symptoms have been found to be highly prevalent across anxiety disorders and to be associated with greater severity and impairment (Ginsburg, Riddle and Davies 2006). Sometimes children and families have not recognized the link between these somatic complaints and the child's anxiety and have instead become worried about possible medical conditions. Children with anxiety can also be overly focussed on what is happening within their bodies. They are quick to notice and focus on feelings that other children readily dismiss. For example, they may be very focussed on any small stomach sensations and can interpret these as a sign that they are going to be sick; or they may notice their heart beating quickly and worry that they will have a heart attack. It is unclear whether children with anxiety actually have greater somatic symptoms on objective measures or whether they worry more about these symptoms than other children do (Kristensen *et al.* 2014).

The increased physical arousal associated with anxiety also can also make settling to sleep difficult. Children frequently report worries around bedtime when their bodies are required to be still and the distractions around them lessen while their minds remain active. Children who worry about upcoming events or who anxiously ruminate on the day are especially vulnerable at this time. This can be particularly challenging for parents who are also tired at the end of the day and are keen to get their children off to sleep. Children with separation anxiety are also likely to have trouble going to sleep without their parents, with sleep representing a lengthy and unpredictable separation.

Difficulties with getting to sleep have been clearly documented in children with anxiety (for a review see Alfano, Gonzalez and Meers 2019). Anxious thoughts in the pre-sleep period is one of the ways in which sleep and anxiety may be connected. It is important to remember, however, that this is a reciprocal relationship, and sleep loss increases anxious arousal, both physiologically and cognitively (Alfano *et al.* 2019). Overtired children tend to be more fragile emotionally, and being overtired means that they often take longer to settle to sleep. Clinically we often see this pattern in anxious children, with anxiety and sleep loss snowballing and increasing the difficulties. Alfano (2018) reviewed the relevant literature to find that there was some evidence to suggest that anxiety-focussed CBT reduced some of the most common sleep complaints for children with anxiety, particularly those that occur around bedtime. Further research is needed; however, this highlights the importance of asking about sleep at the point of assessment and considering interventions that reduce night-time worry and move the child toward getting an appropriate amount of sleep.

It is important to think broadly about somatic symptoms. While stomachaches, headaches and sleep difficulties are among the most common symptoms we see in our clinics, there are a broad range of symptoms that can be associated with anxiety. These include chest pain, dizziness or faintness, excessive tiredness and frequent toileting. Some families describe skin irritations such as eczema as being exacerbated by anxiety. In some instances, medical complaints are the basis of a child's presentation and they will only be referred for therapy when testing fails to identify a medical cause. For these families, an important part of the assessment and therapy is helping them to understand how the symptoms relate to anxiety.

## Cognitive responses

### ALICIA

Alicia (6 years) was described by her parents as always having been sensitive. Her parents made a number of accommodations as a result. For example, when Alicia went to a swimming pool party, they explained that she would not be swimming as she was worried about doing so. They stayed close by her, sitting and watching the other children.

A similar cognitive response is apparent across anxiety disorders, with attentional and interpretation biases often being reported. Attentional bias refers to the tendency of anxious children to focus on threat-relevant information. In practice we see that children with anxiety can often seem to be on the lookout for danger, constantly scanning the environment with wide eyes.

In addition, children with anxiety also tend to display cognitive or interpretation biases around how they evaluate situations. They overestimate how likely it will be that something bad will happen. For example, a child who is going rock climbing with school will overestimate the likelihood that the ropes will break or that they will slip. This tendency to interpret situations negatively has been demonstrated in the research, with a recent meta-analysis finding that children with anxiety tend to interpret ambiguous situations as threatening (Stuijfzand *et al.* 2017). The association was stronger with increasing age, and it was unclear in younger children, as very few studies have been conducted in those younger than 8 years of age.

Children who are anxious also tend to overestimate how bad it will be when the thing they fear occurs. So, returning to the rock-climbing example, rather than being able to reassure themselves that if they slip while rock climbing the safety belt will ensure that they don't fall, an anxious child will assume that a fall is likely to result in them being seriously hurt. They may even believe that a fall is likely to be fatal. The focus on danger applies not only to physical danger but social concerns as well, such as a child looking for clues that peers dislike them, overestimating the likelihood that they will be laughed at and believing this will be a social disaster. Social situations are often ambiguous, and misinterpretations are common in children with social phobia.

Another common cognitive process that we tend to see in children who are anxious is that they underestimate their ability to cope. Ideally we want children to understand that whatever happens they will find a way to manage and will be ok. Often for anxious children, however, this sense of resilience is lacking. Sometimes this may be the result of their experiences and the way in which they and others have responded to their anxiety. Indeed, parents of anxious children also often underestimate their child's ability to cope, like Alicia's parents in the example.

As is apparent from the above, these attentional and cognitive biases are future-focussed and occur in anticipation of, or in the face of, an anxiety-provoking situation. Rumination, however, is another process that we see in children who are anxious, particularly in those with social anxiety. Children who are anxious will sometimes replay situations in their mind, worrying about something they said and how this might have been interpreted.

In cognitive therapy we often talk about "core beliefs," which are simply our beliefs about ourselves, others and the world. These are shaped by our experiences and influence our experience. For example, we may have a belief that others are essentially good which has been formed by some of our early interactions and allows us to be positive about approaching others. For children, their attachment with their parents shapes these beliefs about themselves. Bolton (2005) argues that we don't need to look hard for a child's core beliefs, and that instead we can see them in what parents say about their children. Think, for example, about Alicia and what it might mean for her to be described as sensitive.

## Behavioral responses

### CHLOE

Five-year-old Chloe was referred for therapy in the context of concerns that she was not speaking outside of the family home. At preschool, which was her first experience in an English-speaking environment, Chloe communicated with her teachers by shaking and nodding her head. She had developed a connection with one other little girl, and her teachers observed that this little girl often did things for Chloe, speaking for her when other children and teachers approached her. Chloe's parents described her as an engaging and fun child whose language abilities in her first language seemed age-appropriate and whose English skills were adequate.

We have already covered some of the behavioral responses we see when children are anxious when talking about the fight, flight, freeze response. We spoke briefly about avoidance in the context of the flight response, and we return to it now as avoidance is a core feature of anxiety. This is generally seen quite clearly in the behavior of children who are anxious, as they typically avoid specific situations, places or triggers (like Chloe avoiding speaking outside of the family home). These children may not be able to verbalize their fears, and we may instead see clinginess, tantrums or oppositional behavior as they seek to avoid a feared situation. Avoidance can, however, be more subtle, and is seen in behaviors such as hesitancy, uncertainty, withdrawal or ritualized actions (Rapee 2012). For example, a child who is anxious about being judged negatively by others may hesitate to engage socially, be quiet and careful in conversations, and quietly withdraw from activities that they perceive as challenging. It is also important to recognize that sometimes avoidance can be cognitive. For example, sometimes the child will avoid thinking about the things that make them feel anxious. They may also find it very uncomfortable to acknowledge the anxiety and will avoid talking about the feeling. Parents may similarly avoid acknowledging or talking about anxiety. Avoidance in some form is seen across all anxiety disorders, with the key differences being in the triggers for the avoidance (Carr 2016; Rapee 2012).

Another behavioral response that we commonly see in anxious children involves engaging in safety behaviors. These also serve the purpose of avoidance of the anxiety. Safety behaviors include checking, having strong rituals, doing something in a modified way or excessive reassurance-seeking. Often children involve parents in their safety behaviors. For example, a child who is anxious about monsters might insist on one of her parents checking under her bed before she goes to sleep at night. Safety behaviors can be helpful, and often in therapy we will use these as a way of gradually having a child face their worries. We might, for example, explain that it is important for a parent to stay beside a child who is fearful of water when they first enter the swimming pool. Safety behaviors do, however, become a problem when a child is using these excessively or when they have been unable to decrease their reliance on these over time. For example, it would not be helpful for Alicia to still be attending parties with her parents when she is 10 years of age.

## Understanding children's responses

As should be apparent from the above discussion, the affective, physiological, cognitive and behavioral processes we commonly see in children with anxiety disorders are related and impact one another. It is important to also recognize that the way children experience their anxiety differs. Some children will experience overwhelming bodily sensations and show little awareness of their thought processes when anxious. Others may get very caught up in their minds, losing themselves to their anxious thoughts and showing little awareness of their behaviors or their feelings in this context. Still others will have different patterns. Research has begun to explore whether children with anxiety disorders can be grouped according to some of the features they display. Pearcey *et al.* (2018) identified three subgroups in a large study of clinically anxious 7–12-year-olds: a typically anxious group, a socially anxious group and an avoidant group. Each had a particular pattern of the processes described above. For example, the avoidant group had high levels of avoidance and low levels of threat interpretation, control and negative emotions.

Developing an understanding of the way in which each child and family experiences anxiety is essential as it can guide your therapy, helping you know where to focus your work, both to ensure maximum impact and to help the child and family have a more complete understanding of their anxiety. We talk about assessing anxiety further in Chapter 2. Being aware of these processes in therapy and helping children and families to have different experiences that allow them to have different ways of viewing themselves, others and the world is an essential part of our work.

## Anxiety and behavioral difficulties

### BEN

Ben was an 8-year-old boy who was referred for assistance with chronic generalized anxiety and behavioral difficulties, including significant difficulties with inattention, impulsivity, hyperactivity and defiant behaviors. He was a highly intelligent and academically capable boy, though in both the clinic room and the classroom he was unable to pay attention for more than a few moments. Parent and teacher ratings of attention deficit hyperactivity disorder (ADHD) symptoms were in the extremely high range, and it had been suggested by school staff that a paediatrician be consulted about stimulant medication. Ben's parents were reluctant to consider medication, preferring to address his anxiety first. After three months of therapy treating his anxiety, not only had Ben's anxiety significantly reduced, but so too had his behavioral difficulties. His attention in sessions and in the classroom improved and his hyperactivity and impulsivity decreased.

Anxiety can present in children in very different ways, so much so that their anxiety may be disguised and the child's difficulties misinterpreted. Comorbidity is high between anxiety and behavioral disorders, estimated at about 25% in clinic samples (Carr 2016; Rapee 2012). We frequently see children with anxiety and challenging behaviors, and sometimes their anxiety is not recognized as it can be overshadowed by their behavior.

Anxious children are often referred to therapists for help not with anxiety but with "anger management," sometimes with associated aggressive behaviors. Anger is frequently a secondary emotion in response to anxiety, and difficulties managing anger are a common symptom of anxiety in children. This makes sense when we think about the fight, flight, freeze response that comes with anxiety—the fight can manifest as verbal or physical aggression. Sometimes parents and teachers are unaware of a child's underlying anxiety, and helping them to understand this is very important, as is treating the anxiety. Many of the therapeutic concepts and strategies that are helpful for anxiety are also helpful for anger, such as calming and regulating the body, so in practice these difficulties often resolve together.

Another common presentation of anxiety in children is in oppositional and defiant behaviors. The strong pull of avoidance in anxiety can manifest in a child refusing to do tasks and insisting on being in control to make things as predictable as possible. It can manifest in an anxious response to any demands from parents or teachers, and again the fight, flight, freeze response can display as a child fighting with authority figures or freezing and refusing to comply with their requests. Helping parents and teachers to understand and respond to the anxiety underlying a child's behavioral difficulties is essential.

Childhood anxiety also has the potential for being misdiagnosed as ADHD. Consider the symptoms that overlap between ADHD and anxiety—inattention, hyperactivity and difficulties regulating emotions and behavior are all seen in children with anxiety and can be so significant that they can look like ADHD. To complicate this further, children with ADHD often experience considerable anxiety as a result of their difficulties regulating their behavior, so the two conditions are often comorbid. Careful diagnostic assessment is required here, with the picture sometimes becoming clearer as a child's anxiety improves, as was the case with Ben.

## Working from a transdiagnostic approach

### TOM

Tom was a 10-year-old boy who was described as shy, clingy and introverted from a young age. As a young child, he experienced difficulties separating from his parents to be looked after by a babysitter, and later, to attend preschool. He had many fears, including fears of the dark, animals and strangers. In his early primary school years, Tom was very quiet and reserved, struggling when routines or staff changed, and often having "meltdowns" after he returned home from school in the afternoon. As he progressed through primary school, Tom's worries increasingly focussed on friendships and schoolwork. He experienced stomachaches before school, and sleep difficulties, though he was no longer scared of the dark, animals or strangers and managed separations well.

### SARAH

Sarah was an 11-year-old girl who worried about germs, accidents, the death of her parents, natural disasters and school performance. She was careful about washing her hands well and checking that she and her parents always had their seatbelts on when in the car. Sarah was very focussed on completing her schoolwork perfectly and spent an excessive amount of time on this, frequently checking over her work and tearing it up when she made small mistakes. She also worried a lot about what other people thought about her, ruminating over conversations with peers and worrying that they thought she was weird.

Children often don't fit neatly into the anxiety disorder categories we have discussed. Indeed, they will tend to have symptoms of more than one disorder. In clinical samples, more than half of the children who meet the criteria for an anxiety disorder also meet the criteria for another anxiety disorder, and others will meet criteria for an additional mood disorder (Carr 2016; Rapee 2012; Spence *et al.* 2018). The high rates of comorbidity raise questions about the usefulness of these diagnostic categories.

Another important aspect to keep in mind about anxiety is that it tends to change in form over time. Weems and Costa (2005) found that there were age differences in the expression of anxiety during childhood. For example, younger children were more likely to experience separation anxiety, whereas social anxiety was more prevalent as children moved into adolescence. Anxiety does, however, tend to persist over time (Hudson,

Anagnos and Ingram 2019). Research has begun to explore the different trajectories a child's anxiety takes over the course of their development. For example, Ahlen and Ghaderi's (2019) findings suggest that children may have a low and stable, a moderate and increasing, or a high and decreasing trajectory. As discussed previously, the way in which anxiety presents changes with a child's developmental level; and while the focus of the anxiety changes, the core aspects of anxiety (the affect, cognitions and avoidance) remain the same. This raises more questions about the usefulness of our diagnostic categories.

Further, some children will have significant anxiety and not meet the criteria for an anxiety disorder. For example, a child may be very fearful and avoidant of new situations yet may not meet the criteria for generalized anxiety disorder. Another child may be very anxious about making mistakes and avoid attempting tasks they perceive as difficult in this context. Both of these children will have anxiety that is both impairing and distressing and both are likely to benefit from therapy despite not fitting neatly into one of the *DSM-5* or *ICD-11* anxiety disorders.

The core aspects of anxiety mean that different anxiety disorders tend to be more similar than different. An analysis of treatment approaches for the various disorders also reveals many similarities, and it is generally agreed that the underlying processes in anxiety disorders can be treated with the same intervention. This is one of the pragmatic reasons for the shift toward a transdiagnostic approach to treating anxiety disorders. McEvoy, Nathan and Norton (2009) define transdiagnostic or unified treatments as "those that apply the same underlying treatment principles across mental disorders without tailoring the protocol to specific diagnoses." Many popular treatment packages utilize this approach, such as the Cool Kids program (Rapee *et al.* 2006) and the Friends program (Barrett, 1999). Newby and McKinnon (2019) note that there is now strong evidence for the effectiveness of these programs. For example, Ewing and colleagues (2015) reviewed 20 studies to find that transdiagnostic CBT was an effective treatment for children with anxiety.

Therefore, conceptualizing anxiety more broadly and focussing on the core components of anxiety rather than an approach based on individual diagnostic categories is likely to be useful. For children this has a key advantage, namely that therapy should support them to manage other anxieties they face, either while they are in therapy or in the future. Modular treatments are also increasingly being developed and these allow therapists to choose which parts of an intervention to administer to which children, based on the presenting problems (e.g., Bunge *et al.* 2017).

Our approach focusses on the common processes that occur in children with anxiety, including the core affective, physiological, cognitive and behavioral components, with very few of our activities focussing on a specific anxiety disorder. Rather than adopting a manualized approach, this book is presented more as a modular approach, with therapists encouraged to choose which areas and activities are best suited to the child and family they are working with, adapting these as needed.

# CHAPTER 2

# ASSESSING ANXIOUS CHILDREN

## MAGGIE

Maggie (7 years) came to her first assessment session with her parents, she sat quietly, her body tense, and looked nervously from the therapist to her parents. She shrugged and muttered "don't know" to any questions that were directed at her. When the therapist introduced a drawing activity for the whole family to participate in, she relaxed a little and was able to join in.

Assessment is an essential basis for therapy. Assessment is ongoing, with our understanding of the child and family deepening and growing over time; however, having a good initial understanding is important. Yet assessment is about far more than collecting information. If we don't build a connection with the family, they are unlikely to return to attend therapy sessions, meaning that all of the information the therapist has gathered will be irrelevant. There is an intricate dance that must occur: building trust and providing hope on the one hand and collecting information on the other. Often children and families are anxious about attending the initial assessment session and this adds to the challenge.

Normalizing any anxiety is important at the beginning of the assessment. Letting the family know that most children and parents are nervous when they arrive for the first session can serve this purpose. Providing an introduction that summarizes what will happen in the session is also containing and should reduce the family's anxiety. This can remain flexible; however, it is important that you convey to the family that you will manage the process. For example, we often say something like this:

> Today is about us getting to know each other. I thought we could play a game and talk together for a bit and then I will spend some time alone with you or with your parents. If I spend some time with you on your own, I'll make sure that your parents get some time just with me next session; and if I spend some time with your parents, I'll make sure you and I get some time to play alone next session. At the end of our next session we'll spend some time with everyone together and come up with a bit of a plan.

The box below summarizes some of the basic information that should be collected in the first or second session about the child's anxiety. This includes information about the focus of the child's worry, the history of the worry and how it impacts on their body (somatic symptoms). We also need to think about how a child responds when anxious. Do they freeze, cling to their parents, or respond in anger? We also need to have a good sense of how their parents respond and how they interact around the anxiety. Finally, we need to know if there is anything the child or family does to try to alleviate the worry. For example, this might include the child insisting that the parent stay with them or the parent providing an excessive amount of reassurance. These behaviors can be termed safety behaviors and they are important to know about as they often serve to maintain the child's anxiety. Older children are often able to answer some of these questions themselves. With younger children we generally need to rely more on parent report; however, younger children can often add important information. Observing them during the session also provides a lot of helpful clinical information. Further, ensuring that even children feel actively engaged in this first session is essential for building rapport.

## Aspects of anxiety and useful assessment questions
(Questions for children are listed in italics.)

### FOCUS AND TYPE
*Is there anything you worry about?*

*What things make you feel scared?*

*Tell me some things that [insert child's age]-year-old children worry about.*

*Some children worry about [insert worry]. Is that something you have ever worried about?*

What is it that your child worries about or fears?

Are there other things that your child seems anxious about?

### HISTORY
How long has the worry or fear been a problem?

*When did the worry start being a problem?*

What else was going on in your lives at that time?

Has your child had any other worries in the past?

### SOMATIC SYMPTOMS
*How does your body feel when that happens?*

*If your worries lived in your body, where would they be?*

*Do your worries ever make it hard for you to fall asleep?*

When you look at your child, what is it about their body that lets you know they are worried or scared?

Does your child ever complain of nausea, stomachaches or headaches? Have these been looked into by your doctor and if so what was the outcome?

Does your child complain of other physical symptoms, like dizziness or feeling faint, chest pain, heart racing or difficulties breathing?

**BEHAVIORS AND AVOIDANCE**

What does your child do when they are feeling worried or scared?

*Is there anything that your worries stop you from doing?*

*Does your worry ever get in the way of you doing anything?*

Do your child's worries get in the way of them doing anything they want or need to do?

What would your child do in that situation if they felt really worried?

**SAFETY BEHAVIORS**

*Is there anything you do that helps when you are worried?*

*What makes it easier when you are worried, even a little?*

What do you do when your child is worried?

---

These questions are appropriate for families who identify that their child has some worries or fears. For other families, though, the initial concerns might be about behavior or anger, and you may need to begin with more general questions about the context in which those behaviors occur. Once you have some more information, you can wonder together about whether or not the child is worried about something. This can be quite a shift for some families, so being collaborative and discovering the underlying anxiety together is important.

One aspect that is worth considering during the assessment process is how the child experiences their anxiety. Some children will experience their worry more cognitively, focussing on their worried thoughts, whereas others will show little awareness of their anxiety, responding quickly with anger and aggressive behavior. Still others will feel unwell, complaining of aches and pains, with little awareness of how this might relate to their worried thoughts. Having a good understanding of this can guide the way we approach therapy. For example, a child who gets caught up in an internal battle with their thoughts is likely to benefit from some behavioral strategies that support them to look after themselves while they are experiencing worried thoughts and may provide a useful distraction. On the other hand, a child who expresses their worry through their body is likely to benefit from noticing the situations in which this occurs and beginning to connect with their worried feelings and thoughts.

It is also important to understand the anxiety in the context of the family. One of the most useful questions to ask is who the child reminds a parent of and why. This can elicit information about a family history of anxiety, though it also sometimes provides useful information about the way in which a family perceives and manages anxiety. Asking about anyone else in the family who has worries or is often sad is also useful. Exploring how the anxiety affects other family members is important. Who does the anxiety affect most and why? Who catches the anxiety and how do they respond to this? Some parents will become anxious and upset in response to their child's anxiety, whereas others will become frustrated or angry. Some parents will feel lost as to how to help their child, whereas others will become directive and push their child to face their worries, believing this to be the solution. Frequently, parents will have different approaches and this may add to the tension between them. Understanding how the family responds to, and interacts around, the anxiety is important prior to engaging in therapy.

More generally, we need to understand a child's strengths and weaknesses and have an understanding of where they are at developmentally. Finding out how they are doing at preschool or school and having an understanding of their social interactions as well as their academic development and health is important. We want to have a good understanding of the family, including their values, culture and community, what their lives look like in a practical sense, how they relate to each other and what their attachments are like. We also want to know about the family's expectations for therapy and understand what their goals might be.

Implicit in the above is the need to collect assessment information from multiple sources. Understanding the child's experience of anxiety in the context of their day-to-day lives is crucial, as is understanding how parents understand and manage the anxiety. Questionnaires can be a useful adjunct to clinical interviews, particularly for families who find it difficult to provide a clear description of the child's anxiety in a clinical interview. In addition to clinical interviews with the child and parents it is important to consider other sources of information, such as your observations of the child's play and of family interactions. Having some information from preschool or school is also important in developing an overall picture of the child's difficulties.

De Los Reyes and Makol (2019) is a useful chapter for those who would like further information on assessing anxiety. Stallard (2009) is also a helpful resource and incorporates a chapter on assessment. Manassis (2016) more generally provides a good orientation to assessing children and families using a CBT framework.

## Family assessment

### LEAH AND DAVID

Leah and David had two children who both had autism spectrum disorders and associated emotional and behavioral difficulties. They had little family support, were socially isolated and were experiencing significant financial difficulties. Leah and David both had very different upbringings and tended to parent quite differently, which added to the challenges they faced. They had not previously engaged in therapy; however, they both felt unsure about the process, believing that it was unlikely to be helpful. Many of these factors became apparent at the time of assessment, and this allowed the therapist to talk with the family about some of these challenges and spend more time developing a shared understanding of the difficulties and helping Leah and David to identify one or two small things they could begin to do differently.

The assessment is an ideal time to assess a number of other factors that are relevant to therapy. These include understanding the way in which the family understands, and communicates about, emotions, having a good sense of their relationships and the child's attachment, and knowing how willing they are to engage in therapy. The extent to which families communicate around feelings varies greatly. Some families talk about feelings a lot and there can be concerns about the extent to which they share this information. For example, in some families, parents may share too much information with their children about adult feelings and experiences. In other families, emotions are rarely talked about and are quickly dismissed. Understanding this is important as it helps the therapist to know how much work on feelings and emotional regulation might be indicated. The specific language that the family uses is also important to understand. We try to use the family's language wherever possible, knowing that doing so will support the family to scaffold the work we do in therapy and will support generalization. Some families will talk about worries, whereas others might talk about stress or anxiety. Other families may have their own words for talking about anxiety and it is important to understand what the family mean by the words they use and how this is manifested.

Attachment is an ongoing process and is one that we can assess through asking about the child's early life as well as asking about and observing their current interactions. Both theory and research suggest that an insecure attachment increases children's vulnerability for anxiety, especially when combined with other risk factors. In their review, Esbjørn and colleagues (2012) outlined empirical support for their proposal that both insecure attachment and emotion regulation difficulties are risk factors in the development of childhood anxiety disorders. They present a theoretical model in which the child–parent attachment relationship influences the development of emotion regulation skills, which in turn are needed to manage anxiety-provoking situations. This speaks to the importance of therapists understanding a child's early life and relationships with parents, as well as their emotion regulation skills.

Sometimes people assume that anxiety occurs only in the context of insecure attachment; however, this is not the case. Considering a child's early life as one of the factors that have potentially predisposed a child to developing anxiety is helpful; however, it is important that we don't make assumptions about this. Current attachments are important too and we need to remember that child and parent factors both influence attachment. Parents who have a warm, attuned relationship with their children are likely to be able to engage well in therapy and support their child through this process. For parents who have a more strained or conflictual relationship with their child, there may need to be more work around the relationship and they may need greater support to engage in therapy. Similarly, understanding how parents relate to their children and observing their parenting style is useful. Depending on the family, you may need to learn more about the parents' own families of origin and attachment histories.

Children who have been exposed to more negative life events and more chronic adversities are at a greater risk of developing an anxiety disorder. Many studies have shown an association between negative life events and anxiety in children (e.g., see Kneer *et al.* 2019). It is important to consider, however, the way in which these factors interact for families. For example, some of this might relate to parental anxiety and the role parents play in supporting children through negative life events. Further, it is possible that childhood anxiety places children at greater risk for negative life events. For example, anxious children may engage in unexpected social behavior which may elicit teasing from their peers. A child's experience of an anxiety disorder may also influence the child and parent evaluations of past life events as negative, perhaps due to reporter bias or perhaps due to a heightened vulnerability of the child to the life events (Boer *et al.* 2002). The mechanisms around this risk and the interactions between risk factors may be complex. From a clinical point of view, however, it highlights the need for getting a good sense of the family history, including parental mental health, and understanding parenting practices within the home.

Another important factor to get a sense of is a family's willingness to engage in therapy and, more generally, to change. One way of doing this is to suggest that the family try something different during the assessment session. Often the family's response to this can be telling. Some families will express a willingness to try this, whereas others will move into a "Yeah but…" or a "'We've already tried that" discussion. For families who have previously engaged in therapy there can be a sense of hopelessness and stuckness, and it is often useful during the assessment process to reflect on their previous experiences and get a sense of what they found helpful and unhelpful.

To summarize, the assessment phase is an important opportunity to assess some of the more general factors within the family that are likely to impact on the process of therapy. Doing so allows the therapist to better plan therapy, pitching it so that it is appropriate to the family's needs.

## Managing the assessment process

Often by the time a child comes to therapy there is an urgency the family feels about the need to make things better. Families can feel frustrated by the assessment process and feel anxious about wanting strategies and recommendations. This is understandable; however, unless you collect a reasonable amount of information, it will be difficult for you to provide appropriate intervention. In order to manage this, it is useful to pre-empt this experience for families. How you do this will depend on the context in which you work. You may be able to talk with families prior to the initial session and explain that the first two or so sessions will involve getting to know their child. Alternatively, this may be explained in the pre-appointment paperwork.

It is also important to be realistic about how much assessment you need to complete prior to beginning intervention. Asking a family to provide information for three sessions without giving them any feedback or suggestions about what they might do differently is likely to be frustrating and anxiety-provoking for parents. Giving the family a brief summary of the issues and suggesting something they can do at the end of the first session, with the understanding that you are still getting to know them, is usually helpful and parents often find this containing. Having something to do alleviates some of the anxiety and it can be something simple that is likely to work for most children. Some ideas of what parents might try, even early in the therapy process, are outlined in the box below. We usually try suggesting just one of these ideas early on rather than overwhelming the family with too many. Choose one that fits for the family based on how they are currently managing the anxiety and relating more generally. Providing some brief feedback doesn't mean that you can't go back and collect further information. Indeed, part of your feedback might be that you need to learn more about how the child is managing at school or the like.

---

### Simple ideas for parents early in therapy

Noticing signs that their child is anxious.

Naming the anxiety and empathizing.

Thinking about a similar situation when they also felt worried.

Noticing times when their child seems worried and manages to do it anyway.

Doing something enjoyable with their child each day.

---

How you structure the assessment will depend on your clinical approach as well as the setting and context in which you work. We would recommend that an assessment involves spending some time with the family, some time with the parents and some time with the child. If the child is older, it is often appropriate to have some time alone with them if they are comfortable with this. Collecting some information from preschool or school is also important as teachers see the child in a different setting and will therefore have observations that the parents do not have.

Having a family session, or at least part of a session with the whole family, is a great way of observing the family dynamics first-hand. It often provides an opportunity to observe anxiety within the family and watch how this is managed. It also conveys the importance of family within the therapy process. Inherent in the bringing of a child to therapy is the assumption that the problem lies within the child, and involving the family gently challenges this. It encourages the expectation that the family are central to resolving the problem.

Family sessions are difficult and many therapists avoid them for this reason. Working with a family in the room requires that you manage all of their different developmental levels and perspectives, doing so in a way that enables everyone to feel safe, supported and heard. Providing some hands-on activities is often useful as it gives everyone a focus and keeps children engaged. It allows you to see how the family negotiates a task and takes the focus off the conversation, which may reduce some of the anxiety.

Learning about the family's strengths also helps. Often assessments can be very problem- or deficit-focussed, which can leave a family feeling deflated and hopeless. Being able to draw out a family's strengths helps to balance this and communicates a sense of hopefulness. A strength might be as simple as having made the decision to attend therapy, finding a good school or a sport that really suits their child, or persisting in finding the right therapist for their child. It can be tempting to ask the parent about the child's strengths or what they do well, and often this can be really helpful. It is terrible, however, when a parent is unable to identify anything and the child has the experience of observing this. If a parent comes in spontaneously talking about what a child does well, we might ask directly about strengths with the whole family in the room. If, however, the parent is more focussed on those things the child is finding hard, we would avoid doing so while the child is in the room until we feel more confident about the parents' ability to notice the child's strengths. In the meantime, we can notice and comment on the child's strengths as well as those of the family.

Helping the family to feel hopeful about therapy and what they might be able to change is important. Sometimes the anxiety a child experiences can be overwhelming for a family, particularly if it has gone on for a long time. Knowing that the therapist has seen children with similar difficulties and that therapy is likely to help is important and is worth stating overtly.

## Keeping assessment playful

### AMY

Amy was an 11-year-old with anxiety and an intellectual disability. She was referred for therapy in the context of increasingly unsettled behavior which began around the time that one of her fathers became depressed. Amy's family drawing depicted everyone looking happy and she denied any worries or concerns. When playing with some family dolls, however, Amy enacted a story in which one of the parents was sick and was administered magic medicine by some supportive grandparents. Her spontaneous play conveyed more of her internal world than her conversation ever could and gave the therapist some insight into what she was experiencing.

The assessment phase is one in which the importance of building rapport cannot be overemphasized and finding the balance between connecting and assessing is essential. Having playful assessment activities that are engaging for children yet also provide us with essential assessment information is therefore crucial. Communicating through play is natural for children and having something to do often helps them to feel less anxious.

Drawing and play activities may have a clinical focus, eliciting information about feelings and thoughts; however, non-directed play is also useful. Themes often emerge in a child's spontaneous play. Further, children are often more comfortable talking while they are playing and drawing. For example, research shows that children who are engaged in drawing are more likely to provide clinically relevant information, even if the drawing is not related to the topic being discussed (see Macleod, Gross and Hayne 2013; Woolford *et al.* 2015).

In the assessment process we need to tune into both what a child tells us (the content) as well as what we observe. A child's free play is often very informative. It is useful to notice any themes that emerge in the play as well as the feelings the child is conveying. It is important not to overinterpret the play, and to watch for themes over time, interpreting these in the context of what you know about the child. Children who are anxious will sometimes play out themes around risk or danger, which can be useful to notice in the assessment phase and to monitor for changes as therapy progresses.

In addition to watching for themes it is important to notice how children play. Children who are anxious may be cautious and hesitant in their exploration of toys in the clinic room, waiting for permission to be allowed to play and constantly checking in with the therapist or their parents. They may be hesitant to initiate interaction and may retreat if the therapist expresses an interest in their play. Alternatively, anxious children can be overactive and impulsive, unable to sit still and moving about the room in a chaotic manner. Noticing how the child's play changes over time as they become more comfortable in the therapy room is useful, as is observing how their play changes in response to what is happening in the room. For example, a child may become frenetically engaged in active play as soon as his parents begin to talk about their concerns.

Noticing how the child relates to you in play is also important. Some children will want you to be engaged, whereas others will prefer to play alone. Some may be directive of you in play, whereas others will seek your input and engage in a cooperative manner. How a child plays with you may give you an insight into the way in which they relate to others. It may also give you an insight into their internal world. For example, a child who consistently takes toys from you and excludes you from the play may feel excluded by their peers at school. A child who is particularly controlling of the play may be doing so in an attempt to manage their anxiety.

In terms of directed play and drawing, there are many different ways of encouraging conversation about worries. The following box contains some ideas for directed drawing around anxiety. Puppet play where you enact a worried character is also useful for understanding how the child understands and manages their anxiety. Animal and figurine play can be used in a similar way.

### Drawing ideas for assessing anxious children

Me when I'm worried.

My family when I'm worried.

My body when I'm worried.

My Mom/Dad/etc., when they're worried.

Me when I'm not worried.

My worry as an animal.

My worry as a shape.

My worry as a color.

My worry as the weather.

The things that worry me.

"I just wanna play a game" is a refrain that you may hear in the therapy room. It can be a good reminder that we have slipped into talking therapy and need to offer the child something more developmentally appropriate and fun. There are a number of commercially produced games that can be useful in this context. Alternatively, you might like to make a game with the child in the session. A simple idea is to make a feelings die (a die with a picture of a feeling on each side) and take turns to roll it and talk about a time when you felt that way. Board games are also fun to make, allowing you to personalize the game to match the interests and needs of the child you are working with. In the assessment phase, discussion of feelings might be encouraged by making a simple board game with pictures of different feelings in the spaces, prompting players to remember a time they felt that way, or to describe something that happens when they feel that way. Alternatively, a board game could incorporate "pick-a-card" spaces, with questions about feelings, thoughts and memories. The following box includes some other simple ideas of playful assessment activities.

**Playful assessment ideas**

Decorate balloons or rocks with different feeling faces.

Make masks with different feeling faces.

Make a feelings die.

Make a feelings spinner.

Make feelings faces with modeling clay.

Make a face out of modeling clay and change the expression as you talk about feelings.

The assessment process is anxiety-provoking for many children, but allowing them choice can help them to feel safe. It is important that we don't try to force children to talk when they don't feel ready to do so. This means that whatever game you play there has to be an option not to talk. For example, you might explain that if a child rolls the feeling die and does not want to talk about that feeling, they can choose to roll again. Alternatively, you might offer to share a time when you experienced that feeling or comment on what some of the other children who come and see you might say.

Noticing that a child chooses not to talk about uncomfortable feelings when playing a game is important clinical information. Providing a space in which a child has this choice is also respectful and allows the child to feel secure in the therapeutic relationship. This is particularly important when working with children who have a history of trauma.

During these first sessions it is important that we are sharing too, giving suitable examples of our own feelings. Sharing with children in this way is part of being playful and allows you to engage them in a developmentally appropriate way. In sharing we also provide children with a normalizing experience, supporting them to understand that we all have feelings and that all feelings are important.

Perhaps most importantly, playing is fun. For children who come to therapy the value of having positive experiences and interactions cannot be understated. This is particularly important in the assessment phase in which the enjoyment of playing together supports the development of the therapeutic relationship. Some of the activities in this book provide fun, playful ways to assess anxiety. These include *Worry vs not a worry throw* (page 81), *Catch that feeling* (page 80) and *Feelings creeping up* (page 96).

## Structured interviews and rating scales

Standardized measures can be a useful addition to the assessment process. Sometimes more structured questions or a rating scale provide parents with an opportunity to identify concerns that they might not have been able to find the words to describe in a less structured context. For therapists, questionnaires can ensure a breadth of coverage that is difficult to achieve less formally and is often useful given the high rates of comorbidity we see in childhood anxiety disorders. Standardized measures also provide some normative information, helping to differentiate between developmentally appropriate worries and those that are clinically significant.

Having a sense of severity is also useful as we move into therapy, allowing us to assess whether or not our therapy is working. Some of this information can be obtained during a clinical interview; and having a practical sense of the anxiety, such as knowing how long a child will spend asking for reassurance or how long it takes them to settle to sleep at night, is obviously helpful. When parents are overwhelmed and anxious themselves, it is understandable that they will struggle to report this information accurately, and so standardized measures can be a useful way of tracking progress in this context.

Standardized interviews, such as the *Anxiety Disorders Interview Schedule for DSM IV (ADIS-IV): Child and Parent Versions*, and the *Schedule for Affective Disorders and Schizophrenia for School-Age Children (K-SADS)*, are sometimes used for providing a comprehensive interview. De Los Reyes and Makol (2019) provide a brief overview of these measures.

Broad-based questionnaires often include an internalizing or anxiety scale and can be a useful way of getting an overall sense of the child's emotional and behavioral functioning. The *Behavior Assessment System for Children (BASC 3)* and the *Child Behavior Checklist (CBCL)* are two commonly used examples of comprehensive, broad-based questionnaires. There are parent-rated and teacher-rated scales for both younger and older children, with self-report measures available for older children or youth.

De Los Reyes and Makol (2019) also reviewed a range of anxiety rating scales that are available, including the *Multidimensional Anxiety Scale for Children (MASC)*, the *Screen for Child Anxiety Related Emotional Disorders/Screen for Child Anxiety Related Emotional Disorders-Revised (SCARED-R)* and the *Revised Child Anxiety and Depression Scale (RCADS)*, providing a summary of the reliability and validity of each. Another commonly used rating scale is the *Spence Children's Anxiety Scale (SCAS)*. These rating scales all have parent and child versions and are suitable for children over 7–8 years of age. For younger children, the *Preschool Anxiety Scale (PAS)*, a parent-rated version of the *Spence Children's Anxiety Scale*, is available. Citations for these scales and the other standardized measures discussed above are shown in the box below.

## Some standardized interviews and rating scales for childhood anxiety

### SEMI-STRUCTURED INTERVIEWS

*Anxiety Disorders Interview Schedule for DSM IV (ADIS-IV;* Silverman and Albano 1996).

*Schedule for Affective Disorders and Schizophrenia for School Age Children (K-SADS;* Kaufman et al. 1997).

**BROAD BASED RATING SCALES**

*Behavioral Assessment System for Children (BASC 3*; Reynolds and Kamphaus 2015).

*Child Behavior Checklist (CBCL*; Achenbach and Rescorla 2000, 2001).

**ANXIETY RATING SCALES**

*Multidimensional Anxiety Scale for Children, Second Edition (MASC*; March 2012).

*Screen for Child Anxiety Related Emotional Disorders/Screen for Child Anxiety Related Emotional Disorders-Revised (SCARED-R*; Birmaher *et al.* 1999).

*Revised Child Anxiety and Depression Scales (RCADS*; Chorpita *et al.* 2000; Ebesutani *et al.* 2010).

*Spence Children's Anxiety Scale (SCAS*; Nauta *et al.* 2004; Spence 1998).

*Preschool Anxiety Scale (PAS*; Spence *et al.* 2001).

Choosing a couple of questionnaires that work for your context and the children you see is likely to be helpful. Having an awareness of the psychometric properties of the questionnaires you use is important; using a questionnaire with a number of children also helps you to develop a good sense of the instrument. For example, there may be particular questions that are especially relevant to the children you work with that you can review when scoring. Choosing measures that include both a parent and teacher version is often helpful as it allows you to gather information from multiple sources. It is also important to keep in mind that not all parents will have the literacy skills necessary to complete questionnaires, so being mindful of this is important.

Often having a broad-based questionnaire as well as an anxiety measure is a good combination. This will allow you to quickly gain information about a child's symptoms in comparison to their peers, which you can integrate into the assessment information you have gained from your own observations and interactions with the child, as well as your discussions with parents and teachers. A broad-based measure can be useful in the assessment phase, covering a range of challenges, whereas specific anxiety measures are often briefer and provide a useful way of tracking a child's progress.

Although questionnaires are useful, it is essential that they form only part of our assessment process. Questionnaires provide a measure of severity and can be useful for exploring a broad range of symptoms from the perspectives of different raters. However, they cannot capture the child's personal experience and need to be understood in the context of your clinical observations and the information that you have gathered from the child and family.

## Formulation

All of the information we collect is only valuable if we can use it to develop an understanding of the child's difficulties and put these in context. This process of formulation is influenced by a therapist's training and experience, and often the process of writing a paragraph about how you understand the challenges can help. Johnstone and Dallos (2013) provide a useful guide to formulating from a range of theoretical perspectives, should you want to explore this further.

# CHAPTER 3

# WORKING THERAPEUTICALLY WITH ANXIOUS CHILDREN

### LUNA

When Luna (12 years) presented for therapy, it was apparent that she and her mother had been struggling with her anxiety for a long time. It was just the two of them and there were daily challenges that were exhausting and frustrating for both of them. They found it useful to talk to the therapist in the first session and returned for the second noting some improvements.

Our very first contact with a child and family can be therapeutic if managed well. Assessments help us to develop our understanding of the child's difficulties and share these with the family, allowing us to move more actively into therapy. This chapter describes this process as well as practical considerations around managing anxiety in the therapy room, working with uncertainty and ensuring that children can use what they learn in therapy in their day-to-day lives. We also look at how to work with families and how to modify therapy to take into account developmental needs, including ideas for helping children with developmental difficulties to manage anxiety.

## Anxiety in the therapy room

### NICK

Nick (10 years) and his mother happened to be riding up in the elevator at the same time as the therapist when they came for their appointment one morning. The elevator was crowded and despite Nick appearing calm his mother kept reassuring him that he was ok as the elevator moved upward. She attempted to move closer to him as she reassured him and did not seem comforted by Nick responding that he was ok.

The therapy room is often a microcosm in which the challenges a child and family face in their day-to-day lives play out. Children who are anxious tend to experience anxiety in the therapy room, as do their parents. This can play out in a range of ways, some of which are obvious and some of which are less so. Children who are socially anxious may be reluctant to speak, whereas children who worry about everything being right may become anxious about the drawings or craft they create. More subtly, children who feel anxious about something bad happening may be reluctant to share this, fearing that if they say it, the thing they dread might occur.

Parents will also bring their own anxiety into the therapy space. Many parents of anxious children are also anxious—it's natural for parents to catch their child's anxiety. There may be other reasons why parents feel anxious about the therapy process. Parents may feel anxious about relating to the therapist, worrying about how their parenting may be perceived. They may also worry about how their child is relating to the therapist: they may be concerned that their child is not connecting with the therapist; or conversely, they may worry that their child is becoming too close to the therapist and might share things they don't share at home. Parents may worry about whether the therapist is the right fit or has the necessary skills to support their family, and there may be contextual factors that add to this anxiety, such as the cost of therapy or the stress of fitting appointments into an already busy schedule. Being mindful of what parents may be experiencing and being able to openly discuss these concerns is important.

Therapists too can experience anxiety in the therapy space. Part of this may be in response to the child and family; however, it can also be about the therapist's own anxiety. In engaging in therapy with a family we become part of the system and we can find ourselves responding to the child's anxiety. We might feel anxious in the therapy room as a result, or even feel annoyed or frustrated. Often as therapists our motivation is to help and we may feel frustrated by children who are not ready or able to talk about feelings in the clinic room. We might feel anxious about our interactions with the parents, particularly if they are older than us or if we don't have the experience of being a parent ourselves.

Sometimes our anxiety can be less about how we are relating to the child and family and more about what we bring to the therapy process. For example, one trainee I worked with had the experience of always being the one to make things better, which was a pattern that was apparent in his own family as well as in his romantic relationship. This pattern also played out in therapy, with the trainee frequently overwhelming families with suggestions and feeling anxious when therapy was not progressing quickly. Through supervision the trainee was able to identify these patterns and be mindful of how these impacted on his work with children and families. Tuning into your own feelings is important, and having ongoing supervision with a supervisor who can help you to notice your responses and identify any patterns is essential.

Anxiety in the therapy room is unavoidable and being able to observe and work with those patterns of anxiety can be very useful. Therapy provides a space for gently noticing and reflecting on those patterns and being able to explore different ways of responding. For example, you can gently notice that a parent seems anxious about an upcoming school camp and comment on how the child's affect changed as the parent was discussing camp. You can help a child to notice the changes in their body and behavior and begin to understand that this is a sign of anxiety. For example, you might say, "I'm wondering how you are feeling. All of a sudden your voice got louder and you started speaking faster" or "You looked worried when I talked about you going to the dentist and I'm wondering what sort of thoughts you are having about that." In this way we support the child and/or parent in developing emotional regulation. In noticing and naming their feelings and thoughts they become better able to manage their feelings and reflect upon how this impacts their family.

Noticing your own feelings is also important. For example, you might reflect to the family your experience of feeling like you want to fix things for the child and wonder together about whether that is similar to how the parents feel. Becoming aware of these patterns often frees families up to respond differently. Some families will need more guidance with this than others, however, and together with a family you can explore what it might be like to respond differently.

## Anxiety, uncertainty and play

### LUCY

Lucy (10 years) was a perfectionistic child who frequently became very anxious and angry at home and at school when she made small mistakes. In therapy she became enraged when doing craft activities, losing focus of the purpose of the activity and becoming caught up on a detail about how something looked. Through therapy, Lucy and the therapist were able to identify that she often had a picture in her head of how she wanted something to be and together they began to notice early warning signs that she was becoming anxious when what she created did not match the picture. The therapist was able to help Lucy understand that things not being right was a trigger for her, and they worked on some coping strategies, such as breathing and positive self-talk, that she could use to manage these situations. More generally, Lucy's therapy focussed on helping her tolerate uncertainty and having a flexible approach. Craft activities provided a great vehicle for exploring these patterns in therapy.

### BELINDA

Belinda (12 years) had anxiety, which occurred in the context of her having a very rule-bound and black-and-white way of seeing the world. She had been previously diagnosed with Asperger syndrome. Belinda was initially reluctant to engage in art and craft activities; however, when the therapist presented some mandala coloring pages, she began to color very carefully, staying within the lines. Over time the therapist was able to engage Belinda in a broader range of craft activities, including messy and unstructured tasks, such as free-painting and making slime. Belinda's engagement in these activities paralleled what was happening in her day-to-day life, where she was beginning to experiment with new ways of responding and was relaxing some of her rules around eating.

Clinically, we know that anxious children find it very difficult to tolerate uncertainty. Not knowing how things will go or how they will turn out causes them to feel worried and unsure. Often children will seek reassurance in this context, and parents and other adults will respond by providing lots of information about what will happen, creating the illusion of certainty and reducing the child's anxiety. The reality is, however, that we can never provide absolute certainty. Indeed, if we could, we would never need to feel anxious; nor would we ever feel surprised and experience the joy this brings. Families will vary greatly in how spontaneous or routine-bound they tend to be. Some families have very few routines in place and need support to implement some structure and rules, which often reduces the child's anxiety through creating predictability. Many families of anxious children, however, need support to be able to be more spontaneous as they often have strong routines and plan well in advance.

Intolerance of uncertainty is a concept that has been explored in the research too. Osmanağaoğlu, Cresswell and Dodd (2018) completed a meta-analysis of studies that explored the relationship between anxiety and intolerance of uncertainty in children. As with adults, the 31 studies included in the analysis showed a strong relationship between intolerance of uncertainty and anxiety in children. Children who were able to tolerate higher levels of uncertainty were less likely to be anxious. All but one of these studies was cross-sectional and the relationship does not imply causality. It is likely that children who are anxious become less able to tolerate uncertainty and that intolerance of uncertainty increases anxiety. Therapeutically it is an important concept to explore in the assessment phase and is often a focus of our work.

Often in therapy we work on helping children to manage uncertainty and to cope when things change, are not perfect or don't go the way they thought they would. As with all our therapy goals, this involves work with the child as well as the parents. Our work within the therapy room provides children and families with a space in which they can experience uncertainty in a different way and be supported if they do become anxious. We can work with parents to build their skills in supporting their child outside of therapy in a manner that helps their child to manage some uncertainty.

Play by its very nature involves a lack of certainty. There is no clear outcome and play fosters exploration and experimentation. Play involves creating and making, and some children will view what they have made as imperfect or feel anxious about how what they have made differs from what they envisaged or saw elsewhere. This provides a great opportunity for the child to experience and learn to tolerate a lack of certainty. When we engage in craft or drawing in therapy, we are also modeling that we can have a go and manage when things are less than perfect. Drawing freehand in therapy gives the child a chance to view your less-than-perfect pictures and to notice that you can tolerate these. Describing any worries that you might have about your drawing and any helpful thoughts that help you to manage is a way of extending this. For some children, like Lucy, the focus of your craft activity might be about managing when what you create is not exactly as you planned. Some of the activities in this book aim at helping children to tolerate uncertainty and manage change. These include *Unknown parcel* (page 199), *Measuring change* (page 197) and *Butterfly changes* (page 196).

Parents also play an important role in helping children to manage uncertainty. Helping parents to understand the pattern of reassurance-seeking is often a key intervention in therapy. Encouraging them to provide a predictable frame for children without providing too much reassurance is often helpful. For example, we might encourage a parent to reassure a child by saying that they will be going out for dinner and will have something nice to eat. This does not involve providing a lengthy explanation about which restaurant they will go to and what is on the menu that they might like to order. Providing a consistent frame without too many details is useful for a number of reasons. Importantly, it avoids reinforcing the idea that life is consistently predictable. Things change—the restaurant might be closed or they may not be serving a particular dish. This also allows the child to learn that they cannot know exactly what will happen but it will be ok. More generally, parents can be encouraged to use flexible language, such as "we might," "perhaps" and "maybe" as a way of building in some uncertainty.

There is obviously a balance here between creating predictability and managing uncertainty. It's a balance that you as a therapist need to find in collaboration with the child's parents. Some children will need greater predictability, such as those with autism spectrum disorders and those who have experienced trauma. However, gradually moving to providing a predictable frame and allowing the child to tolerate some uncertainty within that is usually helpful.

## Working within the zone and learning through doing

As mentioned in the Preface, Vygotsky and Piaget have had a strong influence on the way in which we understand and support children. While the implications of their work has arguably been most apparent in education, there are also aspects that are crucial to understand when working with children therapeutically.

Vygotsky's notion of the zone of proximal development is key when working with children. Vygotsky (1986) proposed that what a child can do independently is far less than what they can do with the support of an adult or a more capable peer. He termed the space in-between what a child can do alone and what they can do with support the zone of proximal development. It is the space in which learning occurs and in which a child can be extended beyond their current skill set.

Directed therapy with children clearly involves scaffolding and support. The therapist structures the session to help the child understand and explore therapeutic concepts well beyond their current abilities. Clearly, learning is important. The child has come to therapy for a reason, and what they are able to do on their own is not sufficient for them to manage some of the challenges they are facing. For an anxious child, often this means that their repertoire of strategies to manage anxiety-provoking situations is limited or ineffective. It is essential that the therapist helps the child to evaluate those strategies and learn some new strategies that they can use when faced with the situations that cause them anxiety.

Herein, however, also lies a challenge. The child will be much more able to reflect on strategies within the safe confines of the clinic room than they will in their day-to-day life. Part of this is likely to be about the child's level of anxiety. Therapy is unlikely to elicit the same level of anxiety that they face outside of the clinic room; and the higher a child's level of anxiety, the harder it will be for them to think about their strategies. Importantly though, another part of the challenge relates to the zone of proximal development. Within the clinic room the therapist provides the scaffolding and support that enables a child to think about and challenge their anxiety in a way that they are unable to do without support. What a child will be able to do independently will be less and it is important that both therapists and parents understand this.

Frequently we hear frustrated therapists talking about how a child they are working with is able to list strategies in the room but is not using these in their daily life. Expecting a child to do so is inappropriate and as therapists we need to ensure that we are working in a manner that increases a child's ability to use what they learn in therapy. Scaffolding is a key part of this. In therapy, scaffolding is provided by the therapist; however, in order to make the most use of what they learn in therapy we need to ensure that parents and teachers are providing support for a child in their day-to-day lives. Communication is obviously the first step here. Parents and teachers need to know what you are working on in therapy in order to be able to provide scaffolding for a child. More specifically, they need to know what a child's triggers are likely to be, what early warning signs they can watch for and what strategies they can encourage the child to use. For example, with a child who feels anxious about making mistakes and is a little weaker at maths, you might encourage parents and teachers to pre-empt this when they are giving the child schoolwork or homework. They might be encouraged to say, "Some of these questions are going to be hard. Have a go at them and we can talk about them later." Or for a child who becomes anxious in social situations you might encourage parents and teachers to notice those times when the child steps away from the group and use this as a moment when they could label the anxiety and encourage the child to take a deep breath before stepping back into the group.

Actively involving parents in each session and fostering good communication between parents and teachers is a great way to ensure that children are supported outside of the therapy context and increases the likelihood that they will be more able to use what they have learnt. Ideally, parents are responsible for communicating with their child's teacher as this will establish good working relationships that should persist after you have finished working with the child and family. Some parents are, however, unable to manage this communication, and sometimes ongoing direct communication with teachers is the best way to ensure that a child is well supported at preschool or school. If this is the situation you find yourself in with the children you work with, we would encourage you to gradually try to build the relationship between the parents and the teacher over time.

In each of the activity write-ups in this book you will see a section on how to talk with parents about the activity and what they can do at home to help. The information in this section is also relevant for teachers.

It is also important that parents understand that this is how therapy will likely proceed. Knowing that their child will need support to generalize what they learn in therapy often helps parents to understand their role in the process. It allows them to understand part of your reasoning about involving them in your sessions and may reduce any resistance they have around this. It should also reduce some of the frustration they may experience about the distance between what a child is able to say and do in therapy and how they actually manage in their day-to-day lives.

Another important learning from Vygotsky is that teaching needs to be pitched at the right level in order to best facilitate children's learning. If we only use cognitive strategies with a young child, they are unlikely to be able to use these in their daily life. They are likely to need too much scaffolding in order to use these strategies and, as a result, they are unlikely to be able to generalize this outside of the clinic room. Rather, the focus should be on simple behavioral strategies that they are able to implement for themselves with a little support from their parents and teachers. For this reason, you will see developmental considerations included for each of the activities in this book. We encourage you to think about the child you are working with and choose activities that fit with their developmental level so that you are able to extend them in your work together while still ensuring that they are well placed to use this learning outside of therapy. For those who are interested, Fuggle, Dunsmuir and Curry (2013) talk further about Vygotsky's theory and how this relates to therapy.

The other essential part of helping children to put in place what they learn in therapy is helping a child to regulate. Being able to calm themselves is essential to being able to think about how to respond to and utilize some of what they have learnt in therapy. Some of the activities in this book, such as *Feeling and thinking brain* (page 100) and *Hitting the pause button* (page 134), introduce the concept of the thinking brain and encourage children to calm their bodies so that they can use this part of their brain. Siegel and Bryson (2012) write about the importance of integrating those parts of the brain that help us to think logically with those parts of the brain that drive our big feelings in order to regulate. They note that changing our physical state, for example by moving our bodies, can calm our minds and allow our brains to function in an integrated way. Being able to explain this simply to both children and parents is important.

In addition to working within and understanding the zone of proximal development, it is essential that we work in a way that suits a child's learning style. As discussed, this was one of Piaget's (2000) greatest contributions, namely that children learn through doing. Presenting therapeutic concepts through play enhances a child's capacity to learn and is very much the approach we take within this book. Each of the activities has a hands-on activity or game that supports a child to explore a therapeutic concept. Most children find these activities engaging and the element of fun further supports a child's learning.

## Common processes in families

### LEON

Leon (12 years) had long-standing generalized anxiety. He was particularly fearful at night and insisted on staying in the same room as his mother in the evening. He would only move from one room to another with his arm around his mother's shoulder, leaning heavily on her. Leon was around a foot taller than his mother and it was uncomfortable and awkward for her; however, she had accepted it as an aspect of their day-to-day life.

### RUTH

Ruth was a 9-year-old with an autism spectrum disorder. She found loud noises and social situations anxiety-provoking and was particularly worried about any changes, however small. Ruth's mother was no longer taking her to school and was keeping her at home as much as possible with the view that once she was less anxious she would be better able to deal with those challenges and would be able to attend school again.

Anxiety is incredibly contagious. Parents catch their children's worries; however, children also catch their parent's worries. Again, when we refer to parents, or to mothers or fathers, we mean those who are responsible for caring for the child, and by family we mean those who the child lives with or has close connections with. Consider for a moment the child who watches his mother avoid eye contact with shop assistants, avoids talking to the other parents at school pick-up and feels sick prior to parties. That child is likely to learn that social interaction is something to be feared and avoided. Much of the time this happens without words. The non-verbal nature of the way anxiety is transmitted can be hard for many parents to appreciate. Often parents will talk about how careful they are not to share their own worries and will find the idea that their child may have been affected by these challenging.

Children who have parents with an anxiety disorder are more likely to be anxious, with heritability rates ranging from 30% to 50% (Rapee 2012; Telman *et al.* 2018). Parental anxiety is likely to be related to a number of other factors that have been identified as risk factors for childhood anxiety, including attachment, behavioral inhibition, traumatic or stressful life events, and parenting behaviour, and it may be that these factors mediate the risk for children (Donovan and Spence 2000). The complex interplay between these risk factors, the role of protective factors and what this means for children in practice is something that requires further research. Clinically, it is important that we consider the role that these factors play within the families we work with and support them to build better ways of relating to each other and to the world.

For example, cognitive processes, such as interpretational bias, have been proposed as one of the factors that may mediate the intergenerational transmission of anxiety. There is some research to show that children of parents with anxiety disorders may display similar interpretational biases to their parents. Van Niekerk *et al.* (2018) found that children of parents with panic disorder interpreted ambiguous situations more negatively than children of parents without anxiety disorders. The same pattern was not found for the children of parents with social anxiety disorder, with further research being required. Interestingly, Fliek *et al.* (2019) assessed typically developing children, aged 7–12 years at three time points over the course of a year. Their findings indicated that when children were anxious, parents often modeled more anxiety and interpreted more situations as threatening.

How parents relate to their child around emotions has also been explored, with difficulties with emotional expression found to be related to childhood anxiety. Emotional expressiveness and emotional flexibility, or the ability to move in and out of emotions in a flexible manner, have been two areas that have been explored in the families of children with anxiety. Van der Giessen and Bögels (2018) used an observational study to find that emotional flexibility was lower in the parent–child interactions of children with an anxiety disorder.

Clinically, it makes sense that the way parents relate to their children around emotions is influential and can shape how children experience anxiety. Most parents have had the experience of trying to settle a baby when they are stressed and worried. Babies seem to pick up on their parent's tension despite many whispered words of reassurance. And it doesn't stop once children have language. Despite my many reassuring words about rollercoasters, I am sure my children have picked up on the way my body tenses when we approach one. Helping parents to be aware of their verbal and non-verbal messages is important. From a physiological point of view, anxiety can be stored in the body like a memory, particularly for children who have grown up with difficult early experiences. This is particularly important to explore with parents in instances of developmental trauma.

Sometimes parents who are anxious will communicate this through words, though it may be more subtle. I remember watching a friend's mother telling her that maybe she shouldn't persist with a new job, that it sounded really difficult and didn't seem like it was a good fit for her. It was clear that this mother was anxious about her child attempting this role and was fearful of failure. There was some clear communication around threat in this exchange and also some beliefs about capacity that were implicit in what was being discussed. When communications such as this occur over time, they are likely to add to a child's tendency to view situations as threatening and see themselves as being unable to handle them. Helping parents tune into the underlying messages they are sending their children is often an important part of the clinical work we do.

While further research into the development of anxiety within families would be valuable, it is likely that the effects of anxiety in families are bi-directional. It is understandable that children who grow up with anxious parents are likely to show some anxiety themselves and it is equally likely that parents are highly susceptible to catching their child's anxiety. It is essential that we have a good understanding of parental anxiety and of the way individuals within a family relate around anxiety. Some parents will have had a history of anxiety and had therapy or done a lot of work themselves and may have a good understanding of their feelings, such that the impact on their child is minimized. Other parents may still be beginning to notice their anxiety and to contain this, which is likely to have a greater impact on their children.

It is also important that parents feel they can use their own experiences with anxiety to support their child, rather than feeling guilty about potentially having passed this onto their child. Understanding what happens for a parent when their child is anxious is important and will obviously be influenced by their own experiences and beliefs. Some parents will, for example, jump from the immediate instance of their child not being able to manage to the belief that they will never be able to cope. Sometimes this reflects a parent's own experience. For example, we have worked with families who in those moments when their child is anxious worry that their child will end up just like, for example, their sister who has never worked and is socially isolated as a result of her anxiety. Often the best way to uncover these thought processes is to ask parents about their greatest fear for their child. You can also ask about what goes through their mind in those moments of anxiety. Often this needs to become a focus in therapy with a view to ensuring that parents are best able to manage their child's anxiety in the moment. If a parent is really finding this difficult and it moves beyond the scope of your work with the family, referring the parent for their own therapy may be useful.

Parents often respond to their child's anxiety by being extremely careful and can often feel like they are "walking on eggshells." They do everything they can to avoid upsetting the child. This can include avoiding particular situations, providing a lot of structure and predictability, or engaging in other safety behaviors. For example, the parents of a child with significant separation anxiety may acquiesce to his demands around their presence, even if this means having the child sleep in their bed, always being in the same room as them and delaying starting preschool. Often the walking on eggshells is a pattern that builds gradually over time. It's completely understandable that parents do what they can to make it easier for their children; however, often by the time a child comes to therapy this has reached a problematic level, with parents sometimes going to very extreme lengths to avoid causing their child anxiety, as in the scenario with Leon above. Expressing your surprise in a respectful manner can be a way of alerting the parents to the extent of their safety behaviors and is sometimes the catalyst for change.

Another pattern that often occurs around anxiety is that of excessive reassurance-seeking. Reassurance-seeking involves the child checking with someone in times of anxiety. Typically, they will ask if it will be ok, though children may also ask for details about an upcoming situation or "What will happen if…?" Giving reassurance is a natural part of parenting. It's important that our children seek comfort from us and that we are able to give this to them, so most parents will readily do so. Reassurance-seeking in and of itself if not a problem; however, when children are anxious, this can easily become excessive. In excessive reassurance-seeking the child's anxiety is reduced in the short term when they are provided with reassurance. In the longer term, however, excessive reassurance-seeking contributes to the maintenance of anxiety and reducing this behavior is associated with better outcomes (Rector *et al.* 2019). So, for a child who constantly seeks reassurance that they won't be late to school, their anxiety about being late persists and their unhelpful thoughts about how likely it is they will be late and how bad it would be if they were late remain unchallenged. Perhaps more importantly though, the child never learns that they can be anxious and that this will pass. Indeed, they never learn that they can be anxious and still do what they want and need to do.

The Circle of Security is a useful model for considering the way in which parents relate to children (Hoffman *et al.* 2017; Hoffman *et al.* 2006). The model talks about the twin processes of parents needing to support their child's independence and provide comfort and support. This model is often used to talk about how we relate to our children in those first years of life; however, the twin processes of providing comfort and allowing independence remain relevant throughout a child's life.

Often parents of anxious children hold tightly to their children and don't encourage independence and autonomy. Part of being careful with their child involves them closely supervising and carefully monitoring, which impacts on a child's autonomy and exploration. All of those wonderful experiences, such as going on the big slide, taking the dog for a walk or riding a bike with a friend are avoided. This is particularly concerning when we keep in mind that independence fosters resilience. Parents of anxious children may also struggle with allowing their child to come to them for comfort, responding in anger or misreading their child's cues and providing too much support. They may have a notion about strength and dismiss their child as weak or fragile when they express fear or worry.

Talking with parents about both the process of fostering independence and providing comfort is useful. It also provides an avenue for talking about how a parent's own feelings come into play. For example, I often reflect on being overseas with my daughter who was 5 years old at the time and was attempting some very large monkey bars. I watched anxiously, trying to let her be independent while dealing with my own fear of her falling and needing to get medical assistance in a country where I don't speak the language. She called "Mom" halfway across and I was extremely relieved to be able to help her down. Finding the balance between encouraging independence and providing support is difficult. It's frequently anxiety-provoking and uncomfortable, and as parents we frequently get it wrong. And that's ok. It's about helping parents to understand the complexity of those interactions and know what is useful to aim for. Parents may need support to learn how to sit back and watch and feel ok about letting their child take risks. They may need help to know when to step in and provide comfort.

Parent work is a key component of therapy, and unpacking some of the processes that occur requires some discussion around how parents conceptualize their child's anxiety and the attributions they make around this. As was the case for Ruth above, sometimes parents will assume that their child needs to be less anxious in order to cope and will resist exposing their child to anything anxiety-provoking until you can work together to understand the child's anxiety in a new way. Sometimes a parent's early experiences come into play and it is important to take the time to explore their own family and early life in order to make sense of how they are relating to their child's anxiety.

Being able to talk to a therapist about how we interact with and support our children is very challenging for many parents. Parents may find it hard to acknowledge their challenges and describe some of their interactions honestly, feeling ashamed or embarrassed. We need to create a space in the therapy room that supports parents and helps them to communicate honestly without fear of judgment. Almost all parents love their children and are trying to do their best. Even those parents who have found themselves in a position where they have been emotionally or physically abusive to their children have done so as a result of their own challenges rather than out of a desire to hurt their child. Assuming that parents want the best for their children is a useful stance as a therapist and often enables you to create a culture of acceptance and honest communication, with the understanding that you are both doing your imperfect best to support the child.

Throughout this book you will notice our emphasis on family involvement. There are many good clinical reasons for involving families in therapy: anxiety disorders often run in families and parents can play a role in the onset and maintenance of anxiety disorders (Wei and Kendall 2014). In practice, we see that when parents change the way they respond to their child's anxiety and better manage their own worries, the child's anxiety decreases. We also see that when parents help their children link therapy with their daily lives, children make faster and greater progress.

It is important to acknowledge, however, that the research around parental involvement is inconclusive. Lippert *et al.* (2019) noted that meta-analyses typically don't find significant differences between child- and family-based treatments in terms of outcome. Wei and Kendall (2014) similarly noted the mixed results in regard to whether family-based interventions provided additional benefit to child-focussed interventions, though they noted some evidence suggesting that parent involvement might be beneficial when parents themselves are anxious or when there is a high level of parent–child conflict. Additionally, Manassis *et al.* (2014) found that when parents were actively involved in therapy, children continued to show improvements when followed up one year after treatment. This pattern was not apparent in the other treatment groups and occurred despite there being no significant differences between the treatment groups at the end of treatment. It is plausible that parental involvement may be associated with more subtle changes, such as improvements in communication around emotion, that don't translate to symptom reduction in the short term. Clinically, it makes sense that active parent involvement could help children to integrate therapy into their day-to-day lives, a process that may occur gradually, continuing long after treatment has ceased.

Our understanding of how parental involvement might support therapeutic outcomes for childhood anxiety remains limited and further research is needed (Lippert *et al.* 2019). In the interim, working closely with parents wherever possible is encouraged as is having a good understanding of the patterns that tend to occur in anxious families. In the next section we consider some useful strategies for helping parents to understand anxiety.

## Helping parents understand anxiety

### IVAN

Ivan (12 years) presented with generalized anxiety disorder as well as some separation anxiety, which had been more apparent when he was younger. Evenings were particularly difficult, with Ivan experiencing lots of worries when lying in bed at night, which then became further complicated by him worrying about worrying, and worrying about getting to sleep, and worrying about falling asleep after his parents and having no one in the house to talk to. Ivan's parents were both highly educated professionals and had attended their own therapy over the years for anxiety and mood difficulties. They came to therapy having tried many calming strategies for Ivan and were looking for more suggestions about what they could "do." Through therapy they were able to understand their own anxious desire to prevent Ivan's anxiety and to move away from needing to fix it for him.

Understanding their child's anxiety is often the most useful intervention for parents as it frees them up to respond differently. It is important for parents to understand what anxiety looks like for their child and how they and others respond to it. Often parents benefit from learning about the fight, flight, freeze response as well as excessive reassurance-seeking. Parents need to know about the role avoidance can play and understand any safety behaviors the child is engaging in.

Ideally we want parents to understand that anxiety is a normal emotion—that it is helpful at times, that it comes and goes, and that we can be anxious and still do what we want and need to do. One useful way of talking about this is to talk about Marlin from the well-known Disney movie *Finding Nemo*. Marlin talks about wanting nothing to happen to his son Nemo, and Dory responds with "Well you can't never let anything happen to him. Then nothing would ever happen to him." Her response implies that Nemo might miss out on many opportunities if nothing ever happens to him. Another way to focus parents on how they manage anxiety is to ask them about what message they would most like to give their child in a difficult situation. Often parents will say something like "Whatever happens, you'll be ok" or "You can do it, even though it's hard." Having established what the parent would like to convey, you can then talk about how they would do this. Reflecting what they might need to say as well as how they could communicate this non-verbally is important.

Wagner and Jutton's (2013) model of riding the worry hill is also a useful one to talk about with parents. Although it was developed for children with OCD, the model has broader applicability and the analogy of needing to ride uphill, work hard and keep on going as the anxiety peaks, only to be able to cruise down the other side of the hill once the anxiety has passed, is one that most parents readily understand. The model emphasizes sticking it out until the anxiety passes and this is an important concept for both parents and children. Knowing that they can be anxious and be ok and that they can be anxious and still have a go is essential. Further, the model helps parents understand that it will be necessary for their child to experience some anxiety in the short term if they are going to have less anxiety in the longer term—the more they ride over the hill, the easier it becomes. The parent is not able to take away the experience of the anxiety; while they can provide a good bike and a helmet and make sure the child has had some practice, it is ultimately the child who needs to ride up the hill. Watching your child experience anxiety is very difficult for parents, and being able to talk openly about what this is like is important.

While it might seem tempting to cover all of this in one session and feel that you have ticked off psychoeducation, in reality it doesn't work like that. Parents need time to engage with and understand these concepts in the context of their own child and family. Talking is useful; however, as with children, pairing this with something hands-on often assists a family to understand a concept. There are a number of activities in this book that are useful for helping families to understand anxiety, including *Fight, flight, freeze statues* (page 98) and *My day full of feelings* (page 83). The other activities in this book also have important learning points for parents in understanding the concepts and interventions relevant to their child's anxiety and therapy. Engaging a family in an activity often supports their learning, making the concepts meaningful for them.

It is important to remember that sometimes the parents will be the focus of your activity, particularly if you are working with a younger child or a child with a developmental disability. In these situations an activity can keep the child engaged while you help the parents to understand and explore a new therapeutic concept. For some parents this will be a more acceptable way of engaging in therapy, particularly early on if they feel like their child is the issue and are reluctant to engage in parenting work. It is also practical—many parents of preschool children will not have other care arrangements for their child and it would be inappropriate for children of this age to wait outside. Further, children are often able to take something away from the activity and working all together means that parents are well placed to support their child with that learning. Finally, engaging in activities together is usually a fun experience and that, in and of itself, has some power and utility.

## Developmental considerations

A developmental focus pervades our work with children. Children need therapy that is adapted to suit their level of cognitive, social and emotional development. We are always mindful of where a child is at developmentally and integrate this into our therapy. The following outlines some suggestions about how we do this in practice. Zandt and Barrett (2017) provide further detail for those who are interested.

Gaining a sense of a child's development is not always straightforward. Of course, having a good understanding of typical developmental is essential in this context. However, children who come to therapy often have areas of development they are struggling with. For example, children who present for therapy often have delayed emotional development and many children who present for mental health intervention will have language difficulties.

Further, children with developmental difficulties are more prone to anxiety and you are more likely to see these children in therapy. Sometimes a child's developmental difficulties will not yet be identified, adding to the challenge of understanding their developmental level. For example, the results of a recent meta-analysis suggested around 81% of children with emotional or behavioral disorders had previously unidentified language deficits (Hollo, Wehby and Oliver 2014).

Often therapists have the experience of needing to translate what they have learnt at university to childlike language. Knowing how children and families talk about worries gets easier with time as you see more children. Children often talk about feeling worried or nervous, though language does vary between families. Some children might talk about feeling stressed, sad or scared. Play has an important role in communicating with children, and our activities later in this book provide a way of explaining therapeutic concepts to children and allowing them to explore them. Play is developmentally appropriate for children and provides them with a hands-on experience, which supports their understanding and learning. Play also provides visual supports, which are useful for children who have language difficulties.

When working with children, we also need to be mindful of how much information they can take in. Often therapists are keen to share what they know or anxious to create change and try to cover lots of concepts in a session. For many children, however, one concept in a session is as much as they can take away. They need repetition and reinforcement in order to learn; slowing down the amount of content enables you to provide this. It is also important to remember that when people are anxious they are able to take in less information. For children and parents attending therapy this is another layer and a good reason to further limit the amount of information we cover in sessions. Checking in with the child and family should allow you to assess how much information they have been able to process and adapt this as needed.

Our ability to process information is closely related to our ability to pay attention. Obviously, younger children will have a shorter attention span, as will those with attentional or developmental difficulties. We need to manage a child's attention during the session, keeping them engaged using movement and play. Further, we need to be mindful that anxiety can limit our ability to pay attention. Anxious thoughts can distract us from focussing on what is happening and impact our ability to learn. For younger children, anxiety may be expressed through increased activity, which is likely to make it difficult to focus and take in new information. Similarly, hypervigilance may mean that a child is focussed on noises in the hallway, limiting their ability to focus on what you are talking about. Monitoring a child's attention throughout the session is important. These points are relevant for parents too. Parents will often be anxious about coming to therapy and may also have attentional difficulties. Often, trying to convey one key point in each session is sufficient and is preferable to overloading parents with lots of information, which they are unlikely to be able to pay attention to and recall.

Another key aspect of working with children is helping them to generalize what they learn in therapy to their day-to-day lives, and in doing so we support them to better manage their anxiety. Having sufficient time to understand a concept supports this, as does using play because it engages many aspects of a child's brain and body and is closer to their daily life than sitting and talking. Supporting generalization also requires the involvement of parents and teachers in the therapy. Children need support to practice what they learn in the therapy room in an ongoing way, so working closely with the system around a child is important. For younger children, this usually means having a parent actively involved throughout each session. For older children, this requires some communication with parents each session so that the child is supported to notice, label and better manage their anxiety throughout therapy. Obviously this is a challenge in some settings, such as schools, where you might see the child but only see the parents occasionally. Being creative about how you work with the system around the child is important, so thinking about regular phone calls or emails should help.

Children, especially younger children, tend to benefit most from behavioral strategies. While it is usually useful to include some cognitive strategies, we generally emphasize behavioral strategies as children usually find these most helpful. This means thinking about practical things the child can do, such as telling someone they feel worried, taking some deep breaths, or going and getting a cold drink of water in addition to thinking about noticing thoughts or using positive self-talk.

The nature of the cognitive work that we do with children also needs to be adapted to suit their developmental level. For younger children who are still developing their capacity for inner talk, our cognitive work is likely to be limited to positive self-talk that they can use as private speech spoken aloud. This can be internalized over time, fitting with the development of inner talk, which is increasingly used in middle childhood (Alderson-Day and Fernyhough 2015). For younger children, we choose simple statements that are applicable to a range of situations that they may experience anxiety in, such as "I can do it." For older children, however, we can work around thoughts in a more complex way. Older children can notice their thoughts, can learn that thoughts come and go, can understand that thoughts are only thoughts, can learn to distinguish between helpful and unhelpful thoughts and can challenge their thoughts if they choose to do so.

In general, the younger the child the more of these modifications they need. So, for example, with a preschool child we might engage them in one therapeutic activity in a session, keeping them focussed for 20–30 minutes, before spending the remaining time with the child's parent, discussing how they can support the child at home. As noted previously, you may choose to use an activity with a younger child as a way of explaining a therapeutic concept to their parents while keeping them engaged. Older children can usually stay engaged for longer; however, we would often still limit it to one or two therapeutic activities in a session, using our conversation around the activity to review concepts that we have previously covered and link the learning to the child's worries.

## Modifying therapy for children with developmental difficulties

### MARY

Mary (5 years) was referred by her preschool teacher with a query around selective mutism. She would not speak to anyone at preschool and seemed to avoid the other children. On assessment it was apparent that Mary tended to play alone at home and communicated to request rather than to engage in back-and-forth conversation. Further assessment was undertaken and Mary was diagnosed with an autism spectrum disorder.

### ANDY

Andy (12 years) had an autism spectrum disorder as well as a mild intellectual disability and a language disorder. He came to therapy as he was angry and aggressive, with this typically occurring when he was anxious about a change or someone having a different idea or opinion to him. Andy was an only child and he and his parents loved to stay at home and play video games. As a result, he was rarely challenged at home and most of the concerns were about his behavior at school and in other settings. He had little ability to recognize and express his feelings and became angry as soon as the therapist mentioned feelings. He enjoyed playing board games in sessions and the therapist was able to gradually engage him in therapy by gently commenting on feelings and thoughts as these occurred in the game. Andy was able to talk about some of his thoughts and then began talking about some of his feelings, including being able to tell the therapist that he was annoyed with her.

Children with developmental difficulties have higher rates of mental health difficulties, with anxiety tending the be the most common (e.g., see Whitney *et al.* 2019). Sometimes anxiety can mask a child's other difficulties, and part of our role is to clarify the child's difficulties through careful assessment, as in the example of Mary above. Helping the family to understand how the child's difficulties relate to their anxiety is also essential. Clinically, we often see that children have some awareness of their difficulties and that this causes a level of anxiety. For example, children who find learning difficult often have an awareness that this is harder for them than for other children, which causes anxiety. Anxiety in turn has its own impact. For example, a child who finds social interactions difficult may feel anxious in this context, preferring to play alone as a result and missing out, over time, on developing essential social skills.

Where areas of challenge exist, it is useful to explore a child's feelings about these activities as well as any anxious thoughts they may experience. As children with developmental difficulties may struggle to identify their thoughts and feelings, considering behavioral responses that may indicate anxiety, such as avoidance or aggressive responses, is also helpful. Similarly, where anxiety exists, it is important to explore a child's skill level. For example, if the child is being described as becoming overly active and disruptive during writing time at school, understanding their writing skills is essential. Being able to offer effective therapy for the child's anxiety that takes into account their developmental difficulties is essential for both the child and family. Indeed, a study by Adams, Clark and Simpson (2019) suggested that anxiety was associated with poorer quality of life for children with an autism spectrum disorder.

For children who have developmental difficulties, we often need to make many of the modifications we use for younger children. We reduce and simplify the language we use, slow our pace and provide extra opportunities for repetition and reinforcement. We also actively work on generalization, clearly explaining the links between what we are doing in sessions and their day-to-day lives. Similarly, we work more closely with parents than we would with typically developing children of the same age, knowing that these children will need greater support to put these strategies in place in their daily lives.

Language is key when working with children with developmental difficulties. Having a good sense of their ability to understand language (receptive language) is important as it enables you to pitch your language appropriately. Typically, we gauge a child's understanding of language based on their use of language, so listening carefully to the sentence length they usually use as well as the complexity of their vocabulary and the concepts they can discuss should help. Having a recent language assessment is also likely to be helpful. It is, however, important to be aware that some children's expressive language will be significantly stronger than their receptive language. This pattern is often apparent in children with an autism spectrum disorder, so you will need to be particularly aware of how well these children are understanding. Asking a child to share with a parent what you have talked about often feels quite natural and can be a good way of checking what the child is comprehending.

Similarly, it is important to check in with children with intellectual disabilities and language disorders to ensure that they understand any concepts that you are presenting. Children with mild intellectual disabilities will need therapists to simplify the language they use in therapy. For children with severe intellectual disabilities it is likely to be important to work with the child's parents and school, supporting them to tune into the child's feelings and provide a supportive environment. Working with the child using the activities in this book may not be appropriate as their ability to engage in a language-based therapy is likely to be limited. Other therapies such as music therapy or occupational therapy may be indicated, depending on the child's needs.

Visual supports are a wonderful way of supporting a child's understanding. While this often seems easier with younger children or those who have visual communication systems, thinking broadly about visual supports even with high-functioning children is encouraged. Given the emotional nature of therapy, anything that gives the child another way of understanding what is being said is valuable. Having a sheet of paper or a whiteboard close by so you can, for example, draw the cycle of reassurance-seeking as you talk about it or write some helpful thoughts, is a terrific way of supporting a child's learning. Creating something is another visual support that helps children to understand what is being discussed, as is play.

Children with developmental difficulties often need more opportunities for practice and repetition. In therapy you need to introduce concepts slowly and ensure that you review these ideas in subsequent sessions. Working closely with parents and teachers also gives you greater scope for providing opportunities for practice and repetition. Sending something home with a child at the end of your session and helping parents to know how they might talk with their child about this between sessions is often useful.

Therapy often assumes a knowledge of emotions; however, some children with developmental difficulties will struggle with this. For example, children with an autism spectrum disorder often find it difficult to understand their own feelings as well as those of others. It is important here to differentiate between knowing the name of the feeling and what it looks like in a picture, and understanding what it feels like in our bodies when we have that feeling. Sometimes children will be able to label pictures of emotions; however, they will have very little awareness of what happens to them when they begin to feel anxious. This awareness is essential and ideally we want children to notice smaller feelings or what we might term early warning signs. For example, noticing that you are a little worried and being able to communicate this to a parent or a teacher is by far preferable to letting the anxiety get to the point where you can't cope and end up having a meltdown. Indeed, awareness is often a prerequisite for therapy and can be one of the most useful skills a child learns.

This has important implications for us as therapists. From the outset we need to get a sense of how a child understands their feelings; and where this is an area of challenge, we need to allow time for the child to develop these skills. Many of the activities in this book, including *How does that feeling sound* (page 90), *Hello, it's your body calling* (page 92) and *Fight, flight, freeze statues* (page 98) focus on helping children to connect with the sensations in their body and relate them to how they are feeling. Some of the activities, such as *Feelings creeping up* (page 96), emphasize the need to notice early warning signs and label lower levels of feelings. *Catch that feeling* (page 80) and *Feelings watch* (page 89) can also help children to notice and name their feelings and tune into their experiences, including bodily sensations and early warning signs. For children with an autism spectrum disorder, tuning into their feelings can take time. Having the support of parents and teachers, who can help the child label feelings as they occur, can be invaluable in this regard and reinforces the need for parent work and teacher liaison.

Children with developmental difficulties will often have difficulties with flexible thinking and problem-solving. These executive functions are often challenging for children with an autism spectrum disorder and can also be difficult for children who have cognitive challenges. Often in therapy it helps to decrease the requirement for flexible thinking. For example, when working on helpful thoughts, we might provide a list of helpful thoughts that the child can choose from rather than expect them to generate their own. We may also choose thoughts that are applicable to a number of situations that the child is struggling with, so that they are able to use the same helpful thought in more than one situation. By doing this we are reducing the requirement for flexible thinking.

Similarly, we may focus on getting help from a parent or teacher as a problem-solving strategy with the knowledge that the child will need support to problem-solve and is unlikely to be able to generate appropriate strategies alone.

Another way to reduce the need for flexible thinking is to focus more on behavioral strategies. More generally too, behavioral strategies often work best for children with developmental difficulties. Ensuring that children have things they can do when they are anxious is often helpful, so thinking about behavioral strategies like walking away or getting help, or sensory activities like running around the yard at school, or using a sensory toy, can really help.

Often with children with developmental difficulties we are providing more scaffolding than we would with typically developing children. We do this by using visuals, simplifying our language, reducing the need for flexible thinking, and the like. To return to Vygotsky's zone of proximal development, we provide scaffolding and in doing so create a space in which the child can do more than they can do independently in their day-to-day life. This then raises the question of generalization, which is particularly pertinent for children with developmental difficulties. Children with an autism spectrum disorder, for example, often have a rigid thinking style that makes it hard for them to relate one situation to another. They may, for example, learn that having a break helps when they feel anxious at recess, but they may not think to do this at social events.

As we have mentioned already, within the clinic room therapists can work to support generalization. We can help children to see the relationships between what we are doing in our sessions and their day-to-day lives. For example, when we are using an activity that talks about unhelpful thoughts, we want to make sure that we are drawing on examples from the child's life and relating these to the activity very overtly rather than leaving the child to make these connections. When we hear descriptions of the child's experiences, we can draw these back to what we have talked about in therapy and in doing so support their generalization. Using play also supports generalization. Play is natural for children and is closer to their day-to-day life than working through a worksheet, meaning that the leap between what they learn in therapy and their daily life is smaller.

Ideally, therapists shouldn't be the only ones to provide scaffolding, particularly for children with developmental difficulties. Parents and teachers can prompt, guide and support children to use the strategies they learn in therapy at those times when they need them most. For example, a preschool teacher may offer a suggestion that supports a child to calm their body, or a parent might suggest some words for how a child might be feeling. In doing so they support the child to generalize what they have learnt in the clinic room. Ideally the amount of support (or scaffolding) that we provide children with decreases over time, with the aim of helping the child to manage their anxiety independently. Many children with developmental difficulties, however, will continue to need a level of scaffolding throughout their childhood years. This highlights the importance of creating supportive environments for children through close work with both parents and teachers.

Making therapy developmentally appropriate is a challenge and as therapists we don't always get it right. Watching out for non-verbal cues that a child hasn't understood and trying a simpler explanation is important. Checking that a child has understood is also useful, as is encouraging a collaborative space in which children feel comfortable to ask questions or let you know if they don't understand something. Giving yourself the permission to keep trying until you have achieved a shared understanding is also important.

Many of the activities in this book are appropriate for children with developmental difficulties and will require little modification as they build in visual cues, as well as simple language, practice and repetition. Read the developmental considerations in each activity if you feel that you need some ideas for modifying the activity to make it appropriate to the individual children you see.

# PART II

# KEY INTERVENTIONS AND THERAPEUTIC ACTIVITIES

# CHAPTER 4

# THEORETICAL AND PRACTICAL CONSIDERATIONS

Anxious children experience a range of affective, physiological, cognitive and behavioral processes when they are worried, though these features will vary from child to child. Having a good understanding of the individual child you are working with and the particular way in which their anxiety is experienced is essential when planning therapy. Similarly, having a good understanding of the processes that occur around anxiety within the family is a key factor that informs our decisions about what to focus on in therapy.

As discussed, this speaks to the importance of therapy goals being developed in the context of a thorough assessment and understanding of the child and family. For this reason, rather than presenting a manualized approach, we discuss instead the key therapeutic interventions for anxious children and families, encouraging you to focus on those areas that are useful for the child's particular affective, physiological, cognitive and behavioral processes. This therefore fits with more of a modularized program, requiring you to understand which elements are important for the individual child and family you are working with.

One of the challenges in presenting key interventions is that much of what we know about the effectiveness of therapy with children and adolescents comes from research on treatment packages that combine a number of treatment interventions. As such, we would encourage you to be guided by your understanding of the child's difficulties and to constantly review whether the approach you are using is working.

The following four chapters each cover a key area of intervention, including a discussion of the interventions as well as details of a number of therapeutic activities. First though, we will briefly outline the theory and research underlying these interventions, provide some thoughts about using the activities in practice and explain how to involve parents in this approach.

## Theoretical and empirical basis for key interventions

There are some key interventions that form the basis of our work with children who are anxious. These approaches are based in cognitive behavioural therapy (CBT), including acceptance and commitment therapy (ACT), and incorporate elements of other therapies such as narrative and family therapy.

CBT for anxiety in children typically includes: psychoeducation about anxiety and the link between thoughts, feelings and behavior; interventions aimed at assisting children to recognize anxiety, identify and change anxious thoughts, and build skills in anxiety-management strategies such as relaxation; and graded exposure to feared situations (Bunge *et al.* 2017; Rapee *et al.* 2000). Some programs also include problem-solving, social skills or assertiveness training (e.g., Rapee *et al.* 2000).

There is a good evidence base supporting the efficacy of CBT in treating anxiety in children (James *et al.* 2015; Zhou *et al.* 2019). Many of the studies of children included in these meta-analyses were with children over 8 years of age; however, it is worth noting that Hirshfield-Becker *et al.* (2011) found promising support for the efficacy of CBT in treating anxiety in children under 8 years of age in their review of a small number of studies. Developmentally appropriate adaptations, such as focusing on parent involvement, are important.

What is lacking, however, is support for CBT over other active treatments or treatment as usual (James *et al.* 2015). We also don't have a good sense of which aspects of CBT are most helpful and are only beginning to understand which children are likely to respond best. For example, Newby and McKinnon (2019) note that although children with a primary social anxiety disorder show improvement with transdiagnostic CBT, they do not improve as much as children with other anxiety disorders. This pattern of findings is similar to that observed in standard CBT for specific diagnoses.

Cognitive behavioral play therapy is an adaptation designed to make therapy appropriate for preschool and school-age children (Knell 2015), and many of the activities presented in this book fit well within this model. This method incorporates both structured and unstructured approaches and adapts traditional CBT techniques for use in a play setting. Less structured approaches to play therapy, such as child-centered play therapy, are also supported by empirical research (see Lin and Bratton 2015 for a review).

ACT is a newer cognitive behavioral approach that teaches psychological skills to reduce the impact of uncomfortable thoughts and feelings, by recognizing them as transient experiences that children can notice and accept, letting them come and go without needing to act on them. It also aims to clarify what is really important and meaningful for children and families, and to use that to guide action and motivate trying out new behaviors. For example, Hayes and Ciarrochi (2015) have developed an ACT model and program for youth which modifies concepts to take into account developmental considerations as well as positive psychology concepts. A recent study by Hancock *et al.* (2018) provided evidence that ACT may be an empirically supported treatment option for children with anxiety. The ACT model has intuitive appeal, shows initial promising results with adolescents (Livheim *et al.* 2015; Swain *et al.* 2015) and is likely to be a focus of future research.

Mindfulness is one component of ACT that has become popular with therapists and in schools and some families. Mindfulness is the ability to focus on the present moment, acknowledging and accepting one's feelings, thoughts and sensations. Despite the popularity of this approach, research on the efficacy of mindfulness with children with anxiety remains limited (Maric *et al.* 2019). As such, while we incorporate mindfulness as a component of our work with some children, we integrate this into our other frameworks, such as CBT.

A family systems approach also underpins all of our work with children. We find it essential to understand a child and their anxiety in the context of the family, including the way family members relate to each other and around the anxiety. This approach means we work with parents and family systems to facilitate and support lasting change. Family-based interventions for children with anxiety disorders have empirical support, including family CBT (Carr 2019; Kaslow *et al.* 2012) and systemic therapy (Retzlaff *et al.* 2013).

Another theoretical approach that influences our work is narrative therapy (Cattanach 2008; White and Morgan 2006). Narrative therapy positions problems as separate from people, and assumes that families have many strengths, values and skills that can assist in addressing the problem. This approach includes a focus on the narratives or stories that children and families tell themselves, and incorporates externalizing conversations, play and storytelling. Carr (2014) notes that further research is needed into this approach to establish empirical support. There are certainly aspects of the approach that we find helpful in our work with anxious children, which we outline in Chapter 6.

To summarize, our approach is consistent with cognitive behavioral play therapy, with a child's developmental level constantly informing our work. We focus on families, taking a systemic approach, and our work incorporates aspects of ACT and narrative therapy. In addition, we work closely with colleagues from other disciplines whenever this is in the best interests of the child. This includes working with other allied health professionals such as speech-language pathologists and occupational therapists, and medical professionals such as pediatricians and psychiatrists. Having a multidisciplinary approach is useful for many of the children we see and ensures that the family feels well supported.

## Using therapeutic activities

This section of the book includes many activities that you can use to help children understand and explore therapeutic concepts. Having a good understanding of the child's anxiety is essential to being able to choose appropriate activities, presenting these in a way that fits well for the child and family. We would encourage you to modify the activities as needed, being particularly mindful of the child's developmental level. The section on developmental considerations in each of the activities can help you to think about this. While the general statements in this section will provide some guidance around adapting these activities for younger and older children as well as those with developmental difficulties, it is important that you be guided by your knowledge of the individual child's developmental level, modifying your approach accordingly.

Many of the activities included in this book touch on the same concept, such as noticing feelings. Having different ways of presenting the same concept allows for the child to have an opportunity to practice, reinforcing concepts that have been previously introduced. This crossover also allows the child to have an opportunity to consider the concept from a slightly different approach and in doing so supports the child's familiarity and comfort with the concept, helping them to use it in their everyday life.

The activities are playful in that they involve games, drawing and metaphor. Being playful, however, involves more than using playful activities. More broadly, being playful is an approach, and part of being playful involves giving of yourself. Many of the activities that are included in this book encourage you to provide examples from your own life. From a developmental perspective providing examples helps children understand concepts and supports them to link what they learn in the clinic room with their day-to-day life. Perhaps more importantly though, it normalizes the experience of having feelings and supports a key learning that we want to share with them: namely that all feelings are ok and everyone has feelings. Demonstrating this is far more powerful than simply saying it, and giving examples is a great way to do this.

Often therapists can feel unsure about giving examples and how to do so. We encourage therapists to use genuine examples as these are likely to feel much more authentic. Children tend to engage better when the interactions are authentic and it also means that if they ask questions you won't be at a loss to answer them. Try thinking about some of the examples you could use. These might include "I felt worried that I was going to be late this morning" or "I was frustrated when I realized that someone had used the last of the milk and I couldn't have it on my cereal." Everyday examples such as these often work well with children. They are scenarios that children can often relate to and that therapists are typically comfortable talking about.

Sometimes it is useful to share your experiences on a deeper level too. This is certainly something that is encouraged in ACT. Within the model, however, therapists are encouraged to share only about situations that they have processed and worked through themselves. So, for example, you might share with a child that you used to be really worried about talking to others but you made a big effort to do so because you desperately wanted to make friends. It is important when sharing on that level that the story you are sharing relates to the therapeutic process and that the purpose of sharing is to further a child's or family's understanding. If you are unsure about whether or not something is appropriate to share, checking with your supervisor is worthwhile.

Some therapists will feel more comfortable with a playful approach than others. This may reflect their experiences or stage of life or, even more broadly, their own experience of play as a child. It is important to be aware of your own experiences and think about what feels comfortable for you in your work with children. You may, for example, have a preference for the more structured play activities in this book rather than those that require more creativity. Being aware of your individual preferences will help you to feel comfortable in your work with children and families.

## Using therapeutic activities with parents

Parents will also have their own level of comfort around engaging playfully and being included in therapeutic activities. We advocate throughout this book for working closely with parents and in each of the activities there is a section on how to involve them. It is important that parents understand your rationale around engaging them in therapy and that we are mindful of not asking them to do anything that feels uncomfortable.

Working closely with parents means that we have the opportunity to shape how they respond to their child's anxiety. This often comes up in the context of our discussion around therapeutic activities; however, at other times we will have extended discussion with a parent around a topic. Either way, talking about what parents can do at home is an essential part of our work and forms at least part of each session we have with a family.

As with our general approach to working with families, we work collaboratively, exploring what a family is currently doing and helping them to think about what is and isn't working for them rather than assuming that one technique will work for all families. Providing the space to explore parents' beliefs and experiences is also essential in this space. For example, a parent who cannot tolerate their child experiencing any distress, whether as a result of anxiety or being told "no," is unlikely to follow through with exposure tasks or limit a child's avoidance until this is explored further.

In our work with parents there are a number of areas that tend to come up. These include: how families talk about feelings; how uncomfortable feelings, including anxiety, are viewed; the way in which feelings catch within families; how parents can recognize triggers and early warning signs; what calming strategies are available to the child; how avoidance is managed; and how reassurance is provided. These conversations often begin in the assessment phase and continue throughout therapy, sitting alongside our work with the child and often being illustrated in our therapeutic activities.

Therapy programs often include a separate parent-management training module; however, rather than doing so here, we have opted to include suggestions in each section and after each activity about how you might talk with parents about this. This reflects our belief that parents are essential to the therapy process and our preference for working closely with families throughout therapy.

# CHAPTER 5

# RECOGNIZING AND UNDERSTANDING ANXIETY

Recognizing anxiety requires children to tune into their bodies and thoughts, which can be difficult. It is, however, an important first step. Similarly, understanding anxiety is essential for both children and families and is often therapeutic in and of itself.

## Recognizing and expressing worries and fears

### JAMIE

Jamie has been working with a 7-year-old with anxiety for four sessions now. She feels that the child is not progressing and discusses this in supervision. Jamie explains that she has used breathing and has worked on challenging unhelpful thoughts. She has also done some problem-solving work. When the discussion progresses, it becomes clear that the child has little emotional awareness and does not recognize and label their worried feelings. Together, Jamie and her supervisor work out how they can help the child learn how to notice and name their worries, ensuring that this is established before moving onto strategies for managing the worries.

Being able to recognize and express worries is an important prerequisite to doing further work. When a child is unable to recognize and label their worries, therapy often becomes stuck and the therapist finds they need to return to recognition and labelling as a first step. Sometimes recognizing feelings is difficult for the child because they have not had a language around worries within their family. For example, in some families it is more acceptable to be unwell than it is to be worried. Children develop emotional regulation through co-regulation with their parents. Co-regulation is the process of having your parent notice and name how you are feeling and is particularly important in the 1–3-year-old age range. Having a parent notice and name the feeling helps children to associate what they are experiencing in their bodies with feeling worried. The other important aspect of the co-regulation process is that the child learns that the feeling is ok. They learn that both they and their parent can tolerate the feeling and that their parent is able to support them with the feeling. Siegel and Bryson (2012) provide clear, compassionate strategies for parents that encourage this co-regulation and healthy emotional development.

Children with social and emotional difficulties also find recognizing and expressing worries difficult. Consider, for example, a child with an autism spectrum disorder. Their toddler years may be filled with emotional extremes and they may not express emotions in a typical way, making it difficult for parents to notice and name those feelings. Over the years we have seen many children with an autism spectrum disorder who appear to have a disconnect from their bodies and need support to tune into what they are experiencing in order to be able to label their feelings.

Parents too may have their own reasons for finding it difficult to notice and name their child's emotions. They may be struggling with their own mental health and find it hard to be responsive and attuned with their children. They may also have more long-standing difficulties that make this challenging. This might include not having had a supportive relationship with their own parents or difficulties reading their child's emotions and putting themselves in their child's shoes.

To summarize, learning to notice and name anxiety is difficult for some children and families and will need to be a focus of your early work together. Other children will come in with a rich emotional vocabulary and will readily tell you what they are worried about. Establishing a sense of this at the point of assessment and being able to modify your therapy appropriately is important. A number of the activities in this book are useful for helping children to recognize and articulate their worries. These include *Catch that feeling* (page 80), *Worry vs not a worry throw* (page 81), *My day full of feelings* (page 83), *Feelings chart* (page 87) and *Feelings watch* (page 89).

## Recognizing bodily sensations associated with anxiety

### ANGIE

Angie was a 10-year-old girl with a history of anxiety. She returned to therapy in the context of having been unwell with a stomach virus a few months prior. Angie was very anxious about being sick and was wanting to stay home and keep a bucket beside her anytime she felt any twinge in her stomach. This was making life very difficult and was stressful for both Angie and her family. Therapy focussed on helping her to be able to notice the feelings in her stomach without feeling the need to do anything about them.

### ADAM

Adam (11 years) was a very bright child with significant anxiety, which he typically expressed through anger. He had very little awareness of his own feelings and would escalate quickly, with his parents and teachers being able to identify few early warning signs. He was anxious and angry about attending therapy and escalated any time that feelings were mentioned in the therapy room. Adam liked science, and the therapist engaged him in a series of experiments, including making a sensory putty. The therapist used the putty to help Adam tune into his body. When he squeezed the putty tight, the therapist helped him to notice the muscles in his arms and to realize that his muscles also tightened when he became worried. Adam was able to engage in some conversation in this context and indicated that he often didn't notice what was happening in his body.

Much of what we experience in terms of emotion happens in our bodies. When worried, we experience a broad range of symptoms, from our heart beating faster and our hands shaking right through to headaches and stomachaches. While we all experience different symptoms, we each seem to have our own profile of bodily sensations that we experience when we are anxious. For example, I know that if my shoulders tense I'm feeling a little nervous, and if my jaw begins to hurt this is a sign that anxiety is building further. Being able to recognize your bodily sensations will often mean that you can understand that you are anxious before your mind understands that this is what is happening. Bodily sensations therefore are a key part of being able to notice and name anxiety and it's important to tune children into these.

Some children will come to therapy with very little connection with their bodies and will need support to tune in and understand what their bodies might be telling them. There are a number of activities in this book that support children to better understand their bodily sensations when they are anxious. These include *Fight, flight, freeze statues* (page 98), *How does that feeling sound* (page 90), *Hello, it's your body calling* (page 92) and *Feelings creeping up* (page 96).

Headaches and stomachaches are common in children with anxiety. Sometimes children will come for therapy having had medical investigation that has ruled out any issues. If this is not the case, it is worth the family consulting their doctor to make sure there are not any medical issues that have been overlooked. Often, tracking the occurrence of headaches and stomachaches is useful as there may be patterns that are associated with anxiety. For example, a child may experience stomachaches in the morning when they are feeling anxious about school. It is important that parents understand that just because the pain is anxiety-related doesn't make it any less real. The child is actually physically sore and parents need to respond empathetically while still minimizing avoidance. Ensuring that both children and parents understand what is happening with their pain, and have a plan around how to respond, is essential.

You may also see other children who are overly aware of what is happening in their bodies. They may notice every small jump of their stomach and may leap to the conclusion that this means they are going to be sick. For these children the focus is likely to be more around helping them to know how to respond in these situations and how to remember that these feelings will come and go and need not prevent them from doing things.

One of the most helpful things that we can do in the therapy space is to tune into changes in the child's body, reflecting these back and wondering about how they might be feeling. For example, you might say something like "I just noticed that you frowned then and your shoulders seemed to go higher. I'm wondering if my saying that made you feel worried?" Noticing small changes in this way helps children to become more attuned to their feelings and better understand the link between their bodies and their emotions. It also supports parents who might otherwise struggle to notice their child's early warning signs. Reflecting upon signs you have observed can help parents to better interpret their child's behaviour; and hearing how you respond to this provides a useful model of how they might respond at home.

Simple measures of physiology can be useful in this context. At a very basic level this might involve getting the child to put their hand on their chest and notice how their heart is beating. This is often easy enough for younger children and has the advantage of being something parents and children can do without any equipment. Stethoscopes are relatively inexpensive and can be kept in your clinic room for the purpose of checking heart rate. Older children who have a Fitbit, an Apple Watch or similar may like to track their heartbeat using this. Encouraging the child to notice how their heart rate changes when they jump or jog on the spot for a minute and then check it again after sitting quietly or doing some slow breathing is a good way to start. For children who are under-responsive to their bodies, activities such as this support them to be more mindful. For children who are overly sensitive to changes in their bodies, these activities are useful for helping them understand that there is a whole range of body sensations that are normal.

Once the child is able to tune into their heart rate, you can then move into noticing how their heart rate changes when they are worried. Trying to elicit this in the session by talking about worries or looking at pictures of what the child worries about can be useful, as can having children notice any changes they experience in their heart rate between appointments. Encouraging children to monitor their heart rate during exposure tasks and notice any changes that occur over time is often very helpful.

Another way to support a child to notice their bodily sensations is by doing a version of a body scan, a commonly used mindfulness practice. Explain that it can be useful to pretend that you are in a giant scanner which will carefully move along your body and beep if it notices anything. It is helpful to model this for the child by moving your hands gradually down over your body and making a beeping sound where you notice anything. For example, you might beep over your arm muscles, noticing that they are tight. Once you are done, you can think of a word for how you are feeling and encourage the child to have a go.

To summarize, supporting children to notice bodily changes and understand how these relate to their anxiety is an important aspect of therapy work. It is often essential early in therapy, particularly for those children who are under- or over-responsive to these cues, and continues to be important throughout therapy, helping children to better understand their anxiety and monitor their progress.

## Understanding anxiety and reducing the worry about the worry

### VIVIENNE

Vivienne (8 years) found it helpful to learn that her tearful resistance to going to school each morning was related to the worried thoughts she shared with the therapist about something bad happening when she was away from her dad. She was able to identify that the worry was unhelpful as it was stopping her from spending time with her friends. Vivienne was relieved to hear that lots of other children struggle with worry too and that this was something the therapist could help with.

Psychoeducation is an important part of intervening with children with anxiety. It is important that children have a good understanding of what anxiety is and how they experience it. Beginning to evaluate whether anxiety is helpful or unhelpful is often useful, and most children also benefit from understanding that we all have anxiety and that other children have had similar challenges to them. Instilling hope is essential early in therapy and children often like to know what can help.

The important aspects of what children need to understand about anxiety are listed in the box below. While the box might seem lengthy, in reality these points can often be covered quickly. Further, the extent to which each of these points is covered will vary markedly depending on the child's developmental level. For a young child this might be about understanding that we all have anxiety and knowing what it looks like for them, as in Vivienne's case above.

---

### What to cover in psychoeducation about anxiety

What anxiety is.

What anxiety looks and feels like.

How children tend to respond to anxiety.

How parents tend to respond to anxiety.

When anxiety can be helpful.

When anxiety might be unhelpful.

How common anxiety is.

How anxiety comes and goes again.

What we can do about anxiety.

---

The other thing that the example with Vivienne demonstrates is the importance of personalizing this information to the child. Being able to understand the role that their own feelings play is essential and is not something that can be achieved by providing the child and family with an information sheet or a book.

That said, information sheets may provide a very appropriate adjunct to the discussions you have. Books too, are extremely useful for helping children understand worries when they are paired with some discussion about the individual child's presentation and the family's particular circumstances. There is a lovely normalizing aspect to books, reassuring the child that other children have similar difficulties. The box below provides a list of some of the books we find most useful when helping children to understand worries.

> ### Books for helping children understand anxiety, and worry less about the worry
>
> *Baa! Moo! What Will We Do?* by A. H. Benjamin and Jane Chapman.
>
> *When I'm Feeling Scared* by Trace Moroney.
>
> *When I'm Feeling Nervous* by Trace Moroney.
>
> *I Have a Worry* by Tanya Balcke.
>
> *I Have a Worry Colouring-in Book* by Tanya Balcke.
>
> *The Huge Bag of Worries* by Virginia Ironside (author) and Frank Rodgers (illustrator).
>
> *Hey Warrior* by Karen Young (author) and Norville Dovidonyte (illustrator).
>
> *Hey Awesome* by Karen Young (author) and Norville Dovidonyte (illustrator).
>
> *Is a Worry Worrying You?* by Ferida Wolff and Harriet May Savitz (authors) and Marie Letourneau (illustrator).
>
> *Binnie the Baboon Anxiety and Stress Activity Book: A Therapeutic Story with Creative and CBT Activities to Help Children Aged 5–10 Who Worry* by Dr. Karen Treisman (author) and Sarah Peacock (illustrator).
>
> *What to Do When You Worry Too Much* by Dawn Huebner (author) and Bonnie Matthews (illustrator).

Activities are often useful for helping children to grasp some of these important aspects of psychoeducation. For example, *Feeling and thinking brain* (page 100), *Fight, flight, freeze statues* (page 98), *Helpful vs unhelpful worry throw* (page 106), *Codes* (page 104) and *Worry cloud* (page 108) are all activities that help children develop a better understanding of anxiety.

The act of playing through some of these concepts tends to make them meaningful for families. If there is a key concept that you feel is essential for the child and family to understand, a therapeutic activity is often helpful for facilitating this.

For many children, anxiety about the anxiety is a big part of their presentation, and psychoeducation is particularly important in this regard. In the literature this is often referred to as anxiety sensitivity and it relates to the child's tendency to interpret anxiety symptoms in a catastrophic manner. Anxiety sensitivity is considered subthreshold anxiety and is often associated with the development of anxiety disorders. Although anxiety sensitivity has been researched more in adults, Wauthia *et al.* (2019) found that anxiety sensitivity predicted the presence of anxiety disorders in children.

## Being able to scale and consider the timing of worries

### EMMA

Emma (7 years) became nervous about going to the dentist when her mother mentioned that they had an appointment the following day. She noticed and expressed her worry and she and her mother came up with a plan. On the day of the appointment Emma watched her older sister go first so she could see what would happen. She held her mother's hand while she lay in the chair and managed the appointment well despite her anxiety.

### ISABELLE

Isabelle was an 8-year-old girl with generalized worries. She often projected well into the future, worrying about things such as whether or not she would get into a good university. Part of her therapy involved helping her to work out when was a good time to worry.

As discussed previously, children with anxiety tend to overestimate how likely it is that something bad will happen and also overestimate how bad it will be. Similarly, when children are anxious, they tend not to differentiate between something that causes them a little worry and something that causes them significant anxiety. Noticing small worries is important because if children can notice and deal with smaller worries, this prevents their fears escalating. Part of this seems to be about a child's imagination and their tendency to come up with their own explanations for things they don't understand. A child who doesn't express their concern about the dentist may imagine something far worse than the reality and is likely to become increasingly anxious in the lead-up to the appointment. Worries tend to snowball, so dealing with them as they arise is valuable.

Many children will also experience cumulative worry, with a number of small worries building throughout the day until the child returns home and has a meltdown when they feel safe to do so. Parents of children with an autism spectrum disorder are often very familiar with this pattern. The challenges their children face mean that many of the social, emotional, sensory and cognitive demands of school cause them anxiety; and while children may be able to keep it together at school, this often results in a meltdown at home, in the car or even in the car park. Being able to notice and express some of those small worries means that sometimes teachers and schools are able to make modifications that reduce the child's overall anxiety.

The other important reason for beginning to think about the size of a worry is that not all worries require the same response. A tiny garden spider does not require the response that a large poisonous one does; however, a child who is anxious about spiders is likely to have the same response to both. Children often benefit from learning to pause and engage their thinking brains to be able to think about how big a worry something really is. Traditionally, children are presented with thermometer-like scales; however, there are many ways to help children think about the size of their worries. For young children, it often helps to have them pause, take a breath and show you with your hands how big a worry is. This is also a useful strategy for parents as giving their children something to do often goes some way to containing the parents' own anxiety. Some of the activities in this book are aimed at helping children begin to think about the size of a worry. These include *Another word for...* (page 112) and *Pet worry* (page 102).

Children often also benefit from learning about how the size of their worry might change. Letting children know that their worry will decrease when they have a go at what they are worried about is helpful. Children often benefit from being able to discover this for themselves, and in this way it becomes much more meaningful for them. *Worry shrink ray* (page 193) is an activity that focusses on helping children to identify how their worries change over time.

Another factor that we often want to consider in therapy is the timing of our worries. Often children who are anxious worry well in advance of a situation or event, so much so that parents often avoid sharing their plans. We talked earlier about helping children to evaluate whether a worry is helpful or not, and in a similar manner it is often useful to talk with children about when it would be useful to worry about the situation. For example, Isabelle might decide that she wants to worry about getting a good university place in the last couple of years of school. The activity *When to worry throw* (page 113) can help children explore when it might be useful to worry about specific situations or events.

Thinking about when is a good time to worry is useful for parents too. It is helpful to have dreams and aspirations; however, anxious parents often project well ahead. Sometimes they get so caught up in this that it makes it more difficult for them to manage their child's anxiety. More generally too, it can prevent them from living mindfully and being in the moment.

# Catch that feeling

This is a fun way to get children to notice and name feelings as they occur in the session. It is particularly useful for children who tend to deny that they have any difficult feelings, such as feeling worried or sad. It provides a great opportunity for helping children to identify how they experience feelings in their bodies, their early warning signs, triggers and associated behaviors, and for older children, their thinking patterns.

## What you'll need
You will need a small fishing net, the kind that is readily available from discount stores or fish shops. You might also like to use paper and markers.

## Introducing this activity
Explain that noticing feelings can sometimes be difficult and suggest that you work together to catch them. Suggest that you try to catch the feelings in a net as you are playing today and explain that the child can use the net as well if they notice anyone's feelings change.

Engage the child in play that is likely to elicit a range of feelings. For example, some free play with animals might work well for certain children while a board game might be good for others. Notice when the child's feelings change and rush in an exaggerated way to grab the net and "catch" the feeling. Explain to the child how you knew their feelings had changed. For example, you might say, "I noticed that your lips went tight and your eyebrows went down. Are you feeling angry?" Children will usually laugh at your over-the-top attempt to catch their feeling and this will shift the mood again. It is important to catch any changes in feelings early, because if children are too anxious or angry your response may further escalate them.

Try drawing the feelings that you catch on a sheet of paper so that you have a record of them. Remember to enact some different feelings too, so that the child has a chance to catch some of your feelings.

## What families can do
If families are in the room, they can join in the game in a playful way, which is often fun for children. You and the child can watch out for any changes in their family's feelings and catch those in the net too; and the family may catch some of your feelings or the child's feelings.

You may like to lend the family your net between sessions so that they can catch feelings at home. Alternatively, you can encourage them to use a pretend net, again using this in an exaggerated playful way. It is important to ensure that parents understand that it is essential to do this when they notice early warning signs, rather than when the child is very worried or angry. Parents will often need some explanation around this.

## Developmental considerations
This activity works well with both younger and older children. Older children will be able to engage in more complex conversations around this than younger children or those with developmental difficulties.

# Worry vs not a worry throw

This is a helpful activity to use early in therapy, particularly for children who are finding it hard to talk about their worries. It can help children identify and share what they do and don't worry about.

## What you'll need
You will need some paper and either markers or crayons. You will also need Blu Tack® (poster putty) and a soft ball, or some paper bags and scissors.

## Introducing this activity
Tell the child that everyone has worries and that sometimes it can be hard to talk about these. Suggest you play a game to make it easier. Write "worry" on one piece of paper and "not a worry" on another and stick these on the wall with Blu Tack™, some distance apart. Explain that you will tell the child things that children tend to worry about and they can throw the ball to let you know if this is or isn't a worry for them. A list of childhood worries is included in the printable *Common worries for children template* below.

You can also have the child show you how big their worry is with their hands, how this feels in their body, the thoughts they have or what they do when they have that worry. The questions you ask in this activity will very much depend on the child's ability to reflect on their worries and where you are at in therapy with them. For some children, you will be able to talk about all of these aspects of worry, whereas for others being able to reflect on whether or not that is a worry for them will be sufficient.

If you feel that the child would prefer a tabletop activity, then write "worry" on one paper bag and "not a worry" on another. You can cut out the worries below and ask the child to sort them into the bags, depending on whether or not this is something they worry about. If you do the activity this way, make sure to use the blank pieces of paper too, so that children can add any worries of their own as you work through the activity.

## What families can do
When parents attend the session, they can join in the activity too. If they are not in the room when you complete the activity, it would be helpful to talk with parents about what the child identified as worrying her. At home, the parents might like to continue the discussion by noticing and naming the child's worries, and also noticing things that the child feels confident and comfortable with.

## Developmental considerations
For younger children or those with developmental difficulties you may need to simplify this activity. For example, you could write "yes" and "no" on the paper you stick on the walls, or you could draw a worried face and a calm face. If using the paper bags, you can draw pictures to depict the worries rather than using written words. Having parents in the room and encouraging them to provide examples of when a child might have been worried can also be helpful, particularly for younger children or those with developmental difficulties.

Some children find it difficult to be sure about whether something is clearly a worry or not as it depends on the context, so you might like to add a third category: "sometimes a worry" or "sort-of a worry." This adds complexity to the task, so is more appropriate for older children.

# Common worries for children template

| | | |
|---|---|---|
| Being up high | Other people's dogs | Having someone to play with |
| Other kids not liking me | People thinking I'm dumb | Feeling like I can't stop worrying |
| Making a mistake | Things not being right | Being away from my parents |
| Being away from home | Something bad happening to my family | Something bad happening to me |
| Getting sick | Germs | Not being able to breathe |
| Earthquakes, tsunamis and floods | Vomiting | Schoolwork |
| Burglars or kidnappers | | |
| | | |
| | | |
| | | |

# My day full of feelings

This activity helps children to learn that all feelings are ok and that feelings come and go. It can help them to identify what might trigger feelings of anxiety, and what might help in these situations.

## What you'll need
You will need paper and a pencil or pen for this activity.

## Introducing this activity
Suggest that together you look at how feelings change over the day. Begin by drawing how you are feeling right now on the right side of a sheet of paper. For example, you might draw a happy face to show how you feel about seeing the child. On a separate sheet of paper, you can ask the child to draw how they are feeling.

You can then talk about how each of you felt earlier in the day. For example, on the left side of the paper you might draw a tired face for when you woke up. You can ask the child how they felt when they woke up this morning and to draw that face on their sheet of paper. Talk about what happened next for each of you and how your feelings changed. For example, you might draw an excited face for when one of your own children woke up and talked about how excited they were about the school excursion for that day, and then a worried face for when you thought you might be late due to the traffic, creating a timeline of your feelings over the day. Continue with this process until you have listed all the child's feelings throughout the day. It may look a little like our *example* below (Figure 5.1).

Ask the child what they noticed about their feelings. Talk with them about how the various feelings came and went. Wonder together about how long each feeling lasted and notice how many times in the day their feelings have changed. Notice anything that happened around the time their feelings changed.

You might like to extend the conversations about the feelings and ask the child how they felt in their body or what thoughts they had at those times. You might also like to talk about strategies that help when the child is feeling worried.

## What families can do
If parents are present for the session, it can be useful for them to complete the activity too. Often the experience of doing so is very normalizing and supportive for the child and emphasizes the notion that all feelings are ok and that all feelings come and go. These are also important concepts for parents to understand and can be helpful in promoting an acceptance of feelings and reducing parents' anxiety or frustration with the child's anxiety.

## Developmental considerations
This activity is a simple one that most younger children and those with developmental difficulties can readily participate in with their parents in the room. Having parents present ensures that the key concepts conveyed in this activity—namely that all feelings are ok and all pass—can be reinforced at home. Most older children are also happy to do this. If they have a phone, this could be presented as tracking their mood across the day and recording it on their phone.

FIGURE 5.1 MY DAY FULL OF FEELINGS EXAMPLE

# Sending worries

This activity is helpful for children who are reluctant to talk about their worries and also those who seek excessive reassurance. It can help children find a way of expressing their worries and provide a structure within which they can talk about their worries with others. This structure can also help to contain discussions about worries in families and can be useful for helping to support the child to think about any of their worries that may actually be adult worries.

## What you'll need
You will need some envelopes, a pen or markers, and some strips of paper or cardboard.

## Introducing this activity
Talk with the child about how it is often useful to talk about worries, though it can be difficult to do so. Suggest that together you write down some of the child's worries and work out which ones would be good to talk about and to which people.

Using some envelopes, encourage the child to choose some people who are good to talk to. Explain to the child that each envelope can be for a different person. One might be a parent, another might be the child's teacher, another might be a friend. Most children will also like to make one for the therapist and this can be a good opportunity to talk about your role. Allow the child to decorate each envelope in whatever way they like.

Suggest that the child can list their worries on pieces of card or strips of paper and sort these according to who would be best to talk with about that worry. There may be some worries that the child wants to talk to more than one person about so you may need to write some worries down twice and put these in two envelopes. There may also be some worries that the child doesn't want to talk to anyone about and these may need to be left to one side. There may be opportunities to reflect on whether some of the worries belong to other people—for example, adult worries that can be handed over to a parent.

While completing this activity, discuss what it is like for the child to talk about their worries. Understanding who they talk to, when this typically happens and what this feels like for them is often important. For those children who are reluctant to speak about their worries, this may mean identifying who might be helpful to try talking to. Discuss with the child what it would be like for them to take each envelope and talk with each person about the worries inside.

For those children who seek excessive reassurance around their worries, this activity can provide some structure. You may, for example, allocate a time period for the child to talk about those worries with their parents, leaving any that are not talked about for the next day. Having the worries written down in this manner is often containing for children in a way that simply being told they can talk about it later is not.

## What families can do
Parents can easily engage in this activity when they are present in the session. They may be able to suggest worries they have noticed for the child or they could make envelopes to represent the

people they talk to about their worries. If parents join toward the end of the session you can show them the envelopes then and talk about how to use them.

It is helpful for parents to understand the importance of talking with others about our worries and the role that parents have in helping children to manage their emotions. You might like to suggest that the parent put aside some time to work through an envelope of worries with the child (having a clear idea of when they can do this in the day may be useful). You may like to suggest some helpful ways that parents can talk with the child about the worries and also suggest some questions they might like to ask their child. In families where there has been a pattern of excessive reassurance-seeking, having a clear time frame around these discussions is often helpful.

## Developmental considerations

Younger children are likely to need a parent on hand to support them to reflect upon their worries as well as thinking about who they can talk to. They may prefer to draw rather than write on the envelopes and strips of paper. Similar modifications may be needed for children with developmental difficulties.

# Feelings chart

This activity helps children to talk and learn about feelings, to consider different levels of feelings, and to identify situations in which they may have more than one feeling. It is particularly useful when children have worries that they express through anger. It encourages children to tune into their feelings and provides an alternative way of expressing feelings.

## What you'll need
You'll need popsicle sticks, an envelope, cardboard, Blu Tack® (poster putty) and a marker.

## Introducing this activity
Explain to the child that you are keen to learn more about their feelings and suggest that you make something to help with this. Talk with the child about feelings that they have, writing each feeling on a popsicle stick. Include both uncomfortable and comfortable feelings.

Try to include different levels of feelings—including, for example: unsure, nervous, worried and terrified; or annoyed, frustrated, mad and angry. However, be mindful that this needs to fit with the developmental level of the child. It can be useful to play with the different levels of feelings. For example, you could ask the child to order these from smallest to biggest for worried feelings. You can talk with the child about what it's like when they have these feelings, what they notice in their body and what tends to lead to these feelings.

Place the sticks in an envelope and glue one side of the envelope to a piece of cardboard so that the envelope opening forms a pocket at the bottom of the cardboard, as shown in Figure 5.2 below. Have the child come up with a heading to write at the top of the piece of cardboard (e.g., "I am feeling…") and place some Blu Tack® below this. Allow the child to stick the appropriate feeling underneath.

Talk with the child about how sometimes it might be appropriate to put more than one feeling on the chart and about how sometimes one feeling can be hidden underneath another feeling, such as anxiety being under anger. Talk about some examples of times that you or the child have felt angry because you were worried about something.

## What families can do
If you have parents present in the session, they may like to make their own feelings chart to use alongside their child. Having the parent share some of their own examples can be helpful and normalizing for the child. Otherwise, having a child show them what they have made and providing an explanation about how to use it will be important.

Ideally, families choose a time each day to tune into the child's feelings and choose a word or two for the feelings chart. The child is encouraged to change it at other times too if they notice a change in how they are feeling. Identifying a place in the house where the chart can be positioned is helpful.

Some children will value the space this activity creates and won't feel concerned about being the only one in the family to use a feelings chart. Others, however, may prefer that each family member has a chart of their own.

## Developmental considerations

Younger children or those with developmental difficulties often benefit from having fewer and less sophisticated feelings words. Using pictures on small pieces of cardboard is another good alternative for those children. They may need support from parents to think of a word or picture that fits with how they are feeling when using the feelings chart.

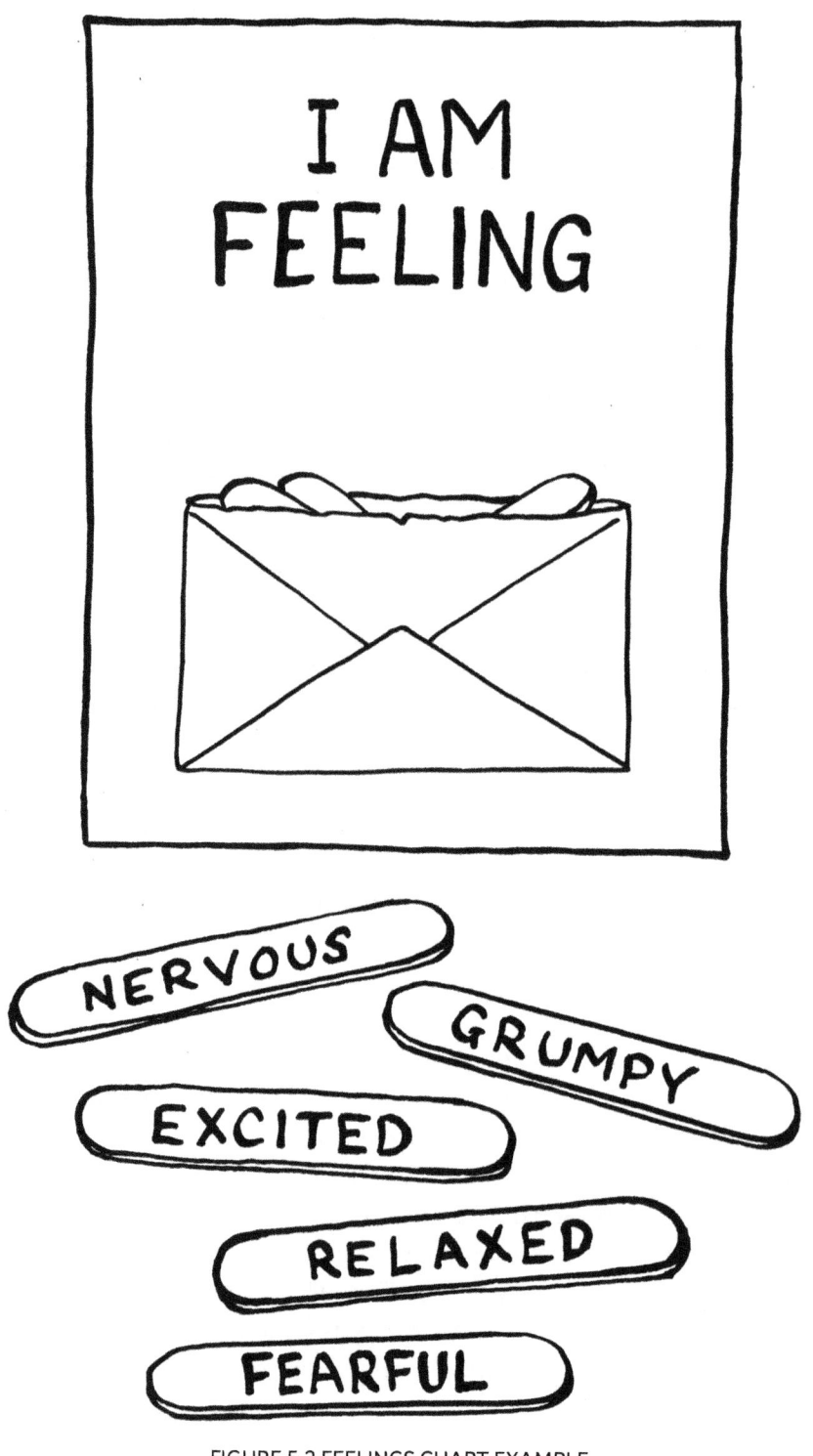

FIGURE 5.2 FEELINGS CHART EXAMPLE

# Feelings watch

Sometimes when children are anxious they struggle to notice their feelings, instead moving quickly into behaviors or focussing on bodily sensations. This activity aims to encourage them to check in, noticing their feelings and behaviors and finding a word for how they are feeling.

## What you'll need
You will need some craft felt, scissors, craft glue, a small piece of velcro and a permanent marker.

## Introducing this activity
Ask the child if they have noticed their parents might check their watches and wonder why they do so. Talk about how we can check our feelings, noticing what is happening in our bodies and our heads. Suggest that you make a feelings watch together to help you remember to check your feelings (see Figure 5.3 below).

First, draw a watch onto the felt using the permanent marker and then cut it out with scissors to create a watch with a band to fit the child's wrist. When drawing the face of the watch, talk with the child about how you can check in with your feelings. Play around with checking the time on the feelings watch, modeling how you can pause and notice bodily sensations and thoughts and think of a word for how you are feeling. Encourage the child to have a go at doing this too.

Glue velcro onto the straps, so you can connect them to fit the watch comfortably around the child's wrist. Talk about when the child might notice their feelings.

## What families can do
Helping parents to tune into their child's feelings and to support their child to notice their own feelings is important. The feelings watch provides a visual reminder and a playful way to encourage this. Parents often benefit from having this modeled in sessions and can provide useful examples about what they notice about their child's behavior and body when they are experiencing feelings.

## Developmental considerations
With younger children a feelings check-in is likely to center more on what they notice in their body or what they tend to do, whereas older children will be able to focus on their thoughts too. Younger children or those with developmental difficulties may find it helpful to have some pictures to choose from when thinking of a word that describes how they are feeling.

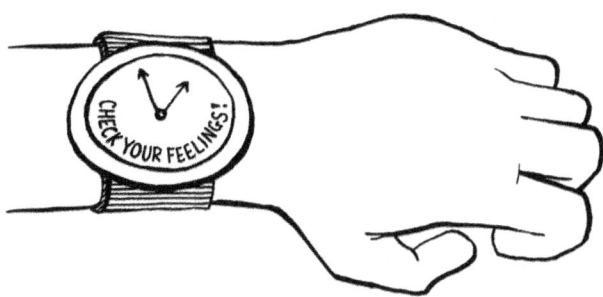

FIGURE 5.3 FEELINGS WATCH EXAMPLE

# How does that feeling sound

This activity helps children explore how they experience different feelings in their body. It normalizes the experience of our feelings impacting on our bodies and helps children to begin identifying the particular pattern of body sensations they experience. This will assist them to notice and understand the physiological changes associated with their anxiety.

## What you'll need

You will need a maraca, a handbell or a tambourine. You will also need a small bell with a hole in the top—you can usually find these in craft stores. You will also need some ribbon or cord to thread through the space in the bell.

## Introducing this activity

Talk with the child about how when we are sad or worried or angry we feel this in our bodies. Suggest that you play a game to understand how these feelings affect our bodies. Ask the child to look away while you act out a feeling while holding the maraca, bell or tambourine and ask them to guess what the feeling is. Exaggerating the feelings will mean that the maraca, handbell or tambourine makes a noise as your body moves and there is likely to be a difference in how the different feelings sound. For example, you might skip lightly to demonstrate feeling happy, which is likely to make a gentler sound; or you might stomp your feet and swing your arms when feeling angry, which is likely to make a louder and faster sound. When the child guesses your feeling, show them what you were doing with your body and describe to them how your body feels when you experience that emotion, noting how tight or loose your muscles are, what different parts of your body do and how your face looks.

You can then ask the child to have a go while you cover your eyes and try to guess the feeling they are enacting. Try to guess when the child has finished and ask questions about what their body is like when they have that particular feeling. Help the child to label the feelings and link them with their facial expressions and body language.

What is important in this activity is not the sound that you make but rather the experience of helping children to connect to their bodies and think about what happens in their bodies when they are feeling worried or experiencing other feelings. Children are unlikely to have the control to manage the maraca, bell or tambourine well and sometimes it will be difficult to guess how they are feeling based on the sound. Guessing and having them show you what they were doing is a good way of getting a sense of the sensations they are noticing in their bodies when they experience feelings.

After you have played a number of times, talk with the child about how it can be helpful to notice what is happening in their body each day and suggest you make a necklace or a bracelet to help with this. Together, thread some ribbon or cord through the small bell and explain that the child can wear this and listen carefully for when it makes a sound, noticing what happens in their body and thinking about how they are feeling.

## What families can do

Parents may like to have a turn of this activity too. This helps to normalize the experience of our bodily sensations and facial expressions changing with our feelings and can be particularly useful if a child is not able to act out different feelings. Children may also be able to act out how parents move when feeling a particular way, which adds to the game-like nature of the activity and sometimes assists parents to develop a greater awareness of their own feelings.

If parents are not present when you complete this activity, you may like to make a short video of the game or audio-record a sound for them to guess at home. Alternatively, encourage the child to take the bell necklace or bracelet home to continue the activity with their family.

## Developmental considerations

Younger children generally understand and engage well with this activity, and most older children enjoy it too. It is particularly well suited to children who prefer to move around the room than sit at a table.

# Hello, it's your body calling

This activity helps children to develop a greater awareness of how they experience anxiety and other feelings within their body and to link these bodily sensations to their feelings. It is particularly helpful for children who are still learning to associate bodily sensations with emotions, and for those who become worried about their bodily sensations.

## What you'll need

You will need markers and a piece of cardboard, a sheet of craft foam or felt, or even a small rectangular box, which you will use to make a phone. You might like to use the *Phone template* below, in which case you'll also need scissors and glue.

## Introducing this activity

Talk with the child and family about how you missed a phone call recently and ask if they ever have this experience. Talk about how this is easy to do, particularly if you have turned your volume right down or are in a very noisy place. Explain that our bodies send us messages too; however, sometimes we are too busy to notice them or don't hear them. Suggest that you make a phone together, so you can think about some of the messages your body might send.

You can make a simple phone together using the cardboard, foam, felt, or box. If you like, you can print the template provided, coloring it in and pasting it onto the phone. Take it in turns to be your body calling with messages, such as "Hello this is your tummy speaking. I'm feeling a little sick. Is something worrying you perhaps?" Sharing some examples of the sensations you notice when your body is calling is often helpful and can be very normalizing for the child. Personalize the play so that you include bodily sensations that the child experiences along with feelings the child often has.

You can ask about when the child finds it easier to get messages from their body and when it might be harder. You can also wonder together about what might be helpful for getting the messages. Would it allow the child to do something differently?

## What families can do

Parents can easily be involved in the session and may provide examples of situations when the child experienced physical symptoms, enabling some discussion about what they might have been feeling at the time. For parents who are not present in the session, when you have completed this activity you can provide them with an explanation and some examples, and have the child show them the phone.

This activity helps parents to understand the link between bodily sensations and emotions. This may assist parents to tune in and hear what their child's body might be saying, supporting them to be better able to label their child's feelings. The child might be happy for parents to use their phone when the child experiences bodily sensations so they can together figure out what their body is trying to say.

## Developmental considerations

Younger children can engage in this activity provided the language remains simple and their parents are present to provide examples of bodily sensations the child might experience and how these relate to their feelings. Having parents continue these conversations at home is also particularly important with this age group. Older children also enjoy this activity and are often better placed to be able to come up with examples of times when they have experienced bodily sensations that link with their feelings. For some children it can be useful to have a list of bodily sensations as examples they can draw on. We have included below a printable list of body changes that are often associated with anxiety.

# Body changes that can happen with anxiety template

| | | |
|---|---|---|
| Feeling hot | Feeling cold | My body shaking |
| Breathing quickly | My heart going fast | Needing to go to the toilet |
| My muscles getting tight or feeling sore | Feeling sweaty | Feeling dizzy |
| Feeling like I'm going to be sick | Feeling like there are butterflies in my tummy | Sore tummy |
| Sore head | Feeling really tired | Feeling like I can't sit still |
| Feeling jumpy | Feeling like it's hard to breathe | My chest feeling tight |

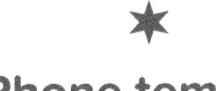

# Phone template

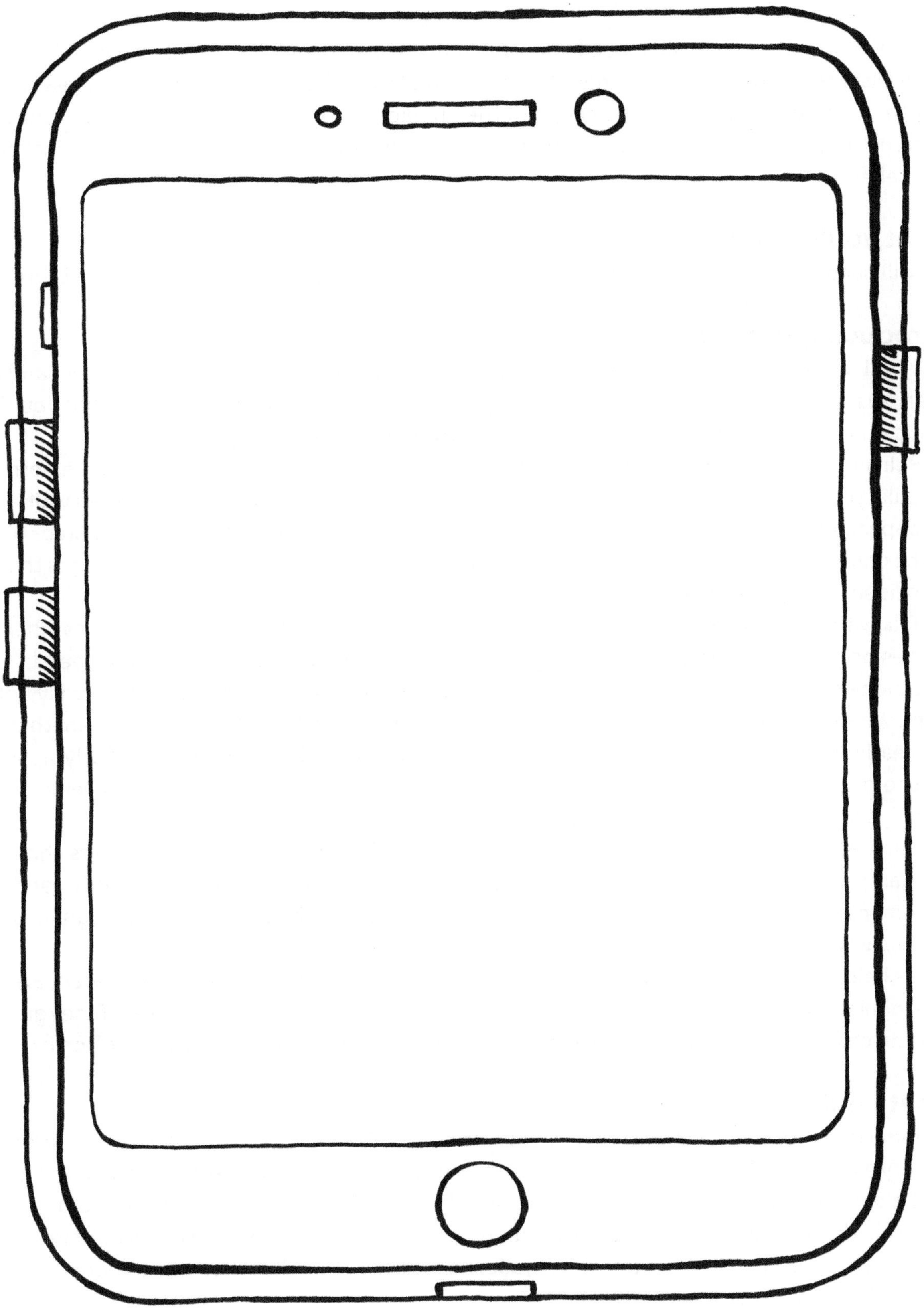

# Feelings creeping up

This activity allows you to talk with children about how their bodies respond when they feel worried and assists them to better track these feelings. It helps children to focus on noticing early signs that they are becoming worried, tuning into their bodies and their thoughts as well as behavioral patterns. It also allows parents to understand their child's early warning signs and tune into these more effectively.

## What you'll need
You will need markers and a long sheet of paper. A roll of craft paper or butcher's paper is ideal.

## Introducing this activity
Explain that you've noticed that sometimes the child's worries seem to creep up on them and that when this happens they seem as though they are suddenly very worried. Suggest that you think about some ways in which you can catch those worries as they are creeping up.

Roll out a long sheet of paper and explain that you are wondering if you can track the worries, a little like you might track an animal by following its footprints. Ask the child if they can walk along the paper and trace their footprints as you do so. You should end up with around six footsteps traced on the paper in a walking pattern. Suggest that you use these footprints to record any signs that the worry is sneaking up on the child.

Talk with the child about what they and their parents have noticed about the times when the worries begin. For example, a parent might notice that a child becomes quiet and spends more time alone or that they seem grumpy, becoming annoyed by things that wouldn't usually bother them. When the child or parent provides an example, encourage them to think about whether that is an early sign or is something that occurs close to the child being really worried. Early signs can be recorded on the first few footsteps, whereas things that occur closer to the child being able to identify that they are worried should go farther along.

You may also like to add in signs that you have noticed, such as a child's movements changing. For example, many children will experience some muscle tightening when they are worried and their movements will become less fluid as a result, or you might see their shoulders rise higher as they become worried.

It's helpful to identify as many early signs as possible so that both the child and parent are able to recognize the pattern more readily. Talking with parents about what would happen if they guessed that the child might be worried and were able to empathize in those early stages is often useful.

## What families can do
Having parents in the room for this activity is ideal. Sometimes the discussion enables parents to identify early signs that they have previously missed. For many busy parents, tuning in at this level can be challenging, so often it is helpful to identify some signs they might see and return to this activity in the next session to give them an opportunity to reflect on what they noticed. Parents may also like to complete their own tracking, modeling for their child that they can recognize some of their early warning signs.

For those parents who aren't present when you complete the activity, you can show them the footsteps afterwards and talk about whether there are other signs that they notice. Discuss how they might notice the early signs when their child is becoming worried at home and how they can support their child in recognizing and managing these.

## Developmental considerations

This activity can be used with younger children; however, having parents in the room is essential when doing so with this age group. Most younger children experience their emotions as very big and overwhelming and they still need parents to help them to regulate. Helping their parents to tune into early signs that they are becoming worried is very helpful and cannot be done without them in the room.

Older children are likely to be able to identify some early signs of their own, particularly if presented with some examples they can reflect on. For example, you may want to utilize the list in the *Body changes* template (page 94). Children with developmental difficulties often find this sort of work easier when they have examples they can choose from.

# Fight, flight, freeze statues

This activity helps children and families understand our body sensations when we are anxious and the ways that we often respond to this. It is a great way to introduce the fight, flight, freeze responses in a way that is meaningful for the child, and provides an opportunity for you to obtain further information about a child's experience of anxiety. It also supports parents to understand some of the behaviors they might be seeing in their children when they are worried.

## What you'll need
You will need a device to play and pause music.

## Introducing this activity
Talk with the child about how most of our feelings occur in our feeling brain. Our feeling brain has an alarm system, the amygdala, and when we sense danger our body gets ready to fight or run away. Alternatively, our body may freeze. Suggest that you play a game of musical statues or freeze dance to explore this. This involves dancing to music and, when the music stops, adopting either a fighting stance (e.g., with fists up), a running pose (e.g., ready to sprint), or freezing mid-dance.

Remind the child that fighting does not always mean physical fighting. Sometimes when we are worried we fight with our words. Similarly, flight is not always about actually running away; sometimes it might be about avoiding a situation.

Eliciting examples as you play about when the child has had a fight, flight or freeze reaction provides an opportunity to obtain further information. Talk about what they noticed in their body at this time and what they did. You may also want to talk about the thoughts they had in these situations. Talking about what the child's typical reaction is feeds nicely into developing intervention strategies.

## What families can do
It is helpful for parents to understand the body sensations associated with anxiety and their child's usual responses to anxiety. This activity can be useful in opening up discussion with parents who might otherwise misinterpret their child's behavior as naughty, and it allows them to better understand what their child's experience is.

Families can easily play this game together in session and it provides a good opportunity to reflect on how other family members tend to respond. If parents join the session later, they may like to participate in a quick round of the game to aid this explanation. If you don't have a parent present when completing this activity, you could take a video of the child playing the game and send this to the parent with an explanation of what the child learnt through the activity. You may like to encourage the family to play the game together at home.

## Developmental considerations
Early primary school children are generally well placed to understand this concept; however, some younger children will most likely find it difficult to understand. Younger children and those with developmental difficulties may, however, still benefit from playing it with their families as a way of

explaining this concept to parents in a meaningful manner. It can also be a useful way of keeping children engaged while you help their parents to understand the concept. Older children still tend to enjoy this activity, particularly if they prefer out-of-seat activities.

# Feeling and thinking brain

This activity helps children understand that their worries occur in their feeling brain and that they are able to pause and engage their thinking brain when managing them. Dan Siegel talks about this concept in a particularly easy-to-understand way with his hand model of the brain. Families often benefit from watching a YouTube clip in which he explains this concept or from reading one of his books (e.g., Siegel and Bryson 2012).

## What you'll need

You will need some air-drying clay or modeling clay. You might like a placemat or other easy to clean surface to work on. A model or a picture of a brain is also helpful. Pictures can be found online or see our simple picture of the *Feeling and thinking brain* (Figure 5.4).

## Introducing this activity

Explain that you've realized how smart the child is and have wondered if they would like to learn more about what happens in the brain when we are worried. Suggest that you make a brain out of clay so you can think about this together.

Using some air-drying clay or other modeling material, help the child to fashion two parts of a brain—a smaller feeling part and a larger thinking part. Make the smaller feeling part of the brain so that it fits underneath the larger thinking part. How well the brain is molded is not important and will obviously vary greatly depending on the child's developmental level and fine motor abilities. The key thing is that the child can identify the two main parts of the brain you want to talk about.

Talk with the child about how the feeling brain and thinking brain interact as you create the brain. For example, you can talk about how when we feel worry in our feeling brain our tendency is either to avoid the situation (flight), or to freeze and not know what to do or to fight (either with our words or our body). Reflect on times when you have had this reaction and ask the child to think about whether they have experienced this. Talk about how our bodies respond and how important our feeling brain is for keeping us safe and helping us to react very quickly when we need to.

Talk about how it's our thinking brain that allows us to make a good choice, like telling someone about the problem or remembering that things will be ok. Reflect on how important our thinking brain is for considering our options, problem-solving and thinking clearly. Reflect on times when the child has been able to use their thinking brain, and also reflect on how they managed to turn on their thinking brain. For example, pausing and breathing often helps children to do this. Naming how they are feeling can also help, as can nurturing from others or sensory strategies that calm the body.

## What families can do

Parents can be involved in the session and talk about times that they notice their child or themselves having feeling brain reactions. They may like to be involved in the modeling process or may prefer to watch and engage in the conversation.

When a parent is not present for this activity, the child can show them the brain they've made after the session and fill them in on what they have learnt about brains, including how helpful both the feeling brain and the thinking brain are. If parents are unable to attend the session, then you may want to email them a YouTube clip of Dan Siegel talking about the role of the thinking or "upstairs" brain.

This activity provides an opportunity to help parents better understand the fight, flight, freeze response, which is particularly important if they are viewing their child's behavior in a negative light without understanding the underlying anxiety. It can also be helpful to reflect with parents on the importance of calming the child's body before talking with them about the worry or expecting them to reason or problem-solve. Parents may be able to coach their children at home by encouraging them to pause and breathe and use their thinking brain.

## Developmental considerations

Most children really enjoy modeling with clay, and the simplicity of talking about the brain as having two parts means that this activity can be accessible for younger children as well as those with developmental difficulties. For older children or those who particularly like science, you may like to add in further details about the brain. You may also find that learning about the brain lends credibility to the work you are doing with them.

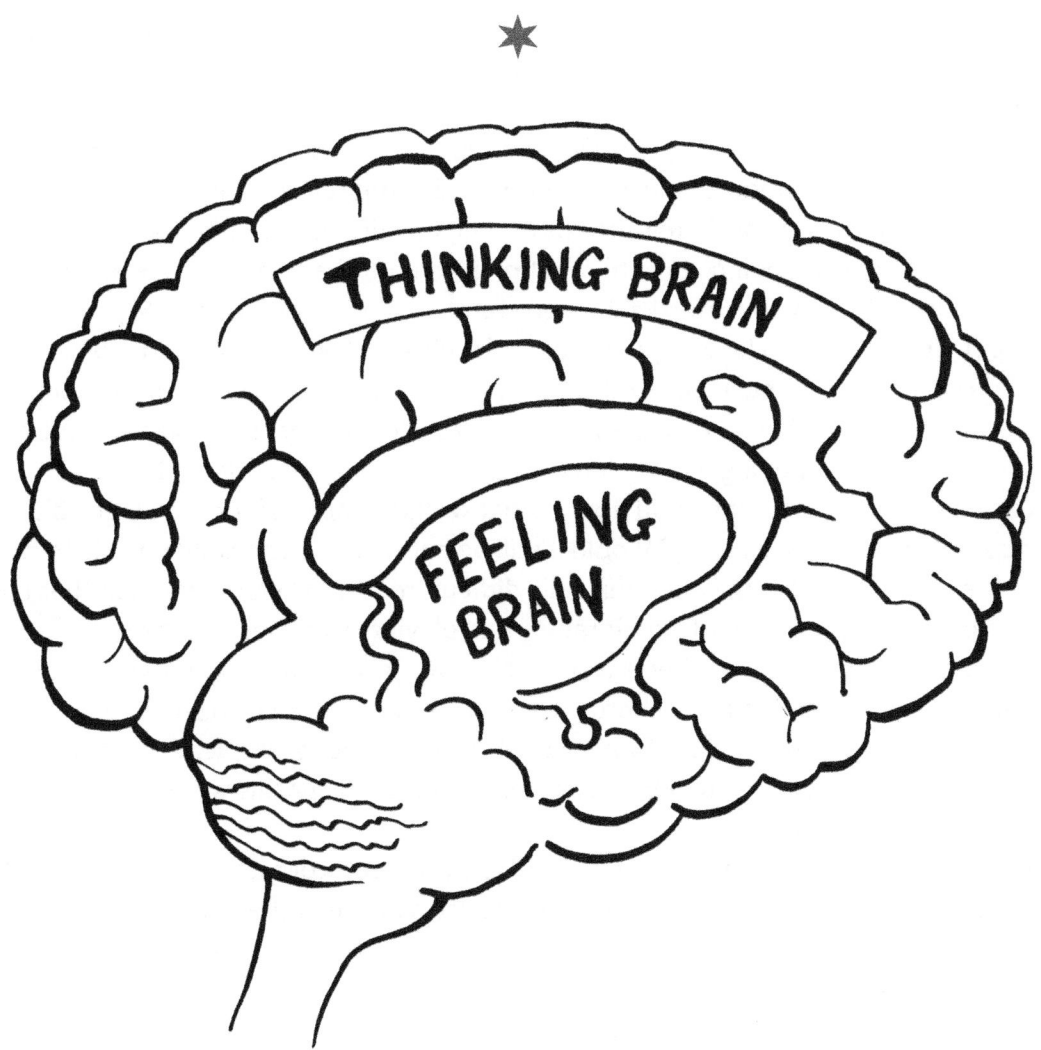

FIGURE 5.4 FEELING AND THINKING BRAIN EXAMPLE

# Pet worry

Therapists sometimes use pet worries in their work with children. This activity uses pet worries to help children understand that a little worry can sometimes be helpful, though focussing too much on worries causes them to grow and become unhelpful. The activity is great to use with children once they have some understanding of how worries work.

## What you'll need
You will need craft materials, including pom poms, googly eyes and craft glue. Additional optional materials are a piece of felt or a popsicle stick, sequins or a permanent marker.

## Introducing this activity
Explain that you've noticed that sometimes the child has a little worry and that this can be helpful in some situations. For example, a child might have mentioned that they were a little worried about going on the flying fox (zip-line) and as a result they were careful to hold on tight. Check with the child about whether or not they thought this worry was helpful and why. Wonder together about what would have happened if the worry got too big. For example, would this have meant that the child would have refused to go on the flying fox?

Suggest that you make a little pet worry to help you think about how the size of a worry changes, whether it is helpful or unhelpful. Using a pom pom, add googly eyes using some craft glue to make a little pet worry. You can add other features by adding bits of felt and sequins or drawing these on with a permanent marker. Adding some felt feet or even part of a popsicle stick as a base is a good way to steady the pet worry, ensuring that it can stand up alone (see Figure 5.5).

These pet worries tend to look cute because of their size. You can talk about what a good size they are. The child is still so much bigger than the pet worry and could put it in their pocket and zip it closed if they needed to. It would be easy to talk calmly to a worry of this size and the child could easily see what else is happening as the worry would not take up all of their vision.

You can then wonder with the child about what would happen if the worry got big. What if it was the size of a three-story building? Would it still be cute? Would the child be able to stop it from getting in the way or would it make things really difficult for them? Would it mean that it would be hard for the child to enjoy being with their family and playing with their friends?

Ask the child if they know what helps worries to grow. Talk about how thinking about worries a lot often makes them bigger and how sharing them with someone else often shrinks them. Bring in other aspects that have been a focus of your therapy together. For example, if you have been talking with the child about using their thinking brain, ask about whether this would help them to shrink their pet worry.

Talk with the child about what size they would like their pet worry to be and ask how they think they can keep it at this size. Together, try to identify ways in which the child might be able to keep the pet worry at a manageable size.

## What families can do

Parents can be involved in the session and may like to make a pet worry of their own, reflecting on how they keep it at a good size. If parents are not present when you complete this activity, the child can show their parents the pet worry and together discuss their plans to keep it small and how the parents can help with this.

It is important for parents to understand how worries can be helpful or unhelpful, and how the size of the worry can relate to this. Parents can continue these conversations at home and may be able to notice when their child's pet worry seems small and cute, and when it seems to be growing or getting in the way.

## Developmental considerations

Older children are better placed to understand some of the concepts discussed in this activity. For many younger children some of this will be too abstract and the imagery of their worries as a big monster may be scary.

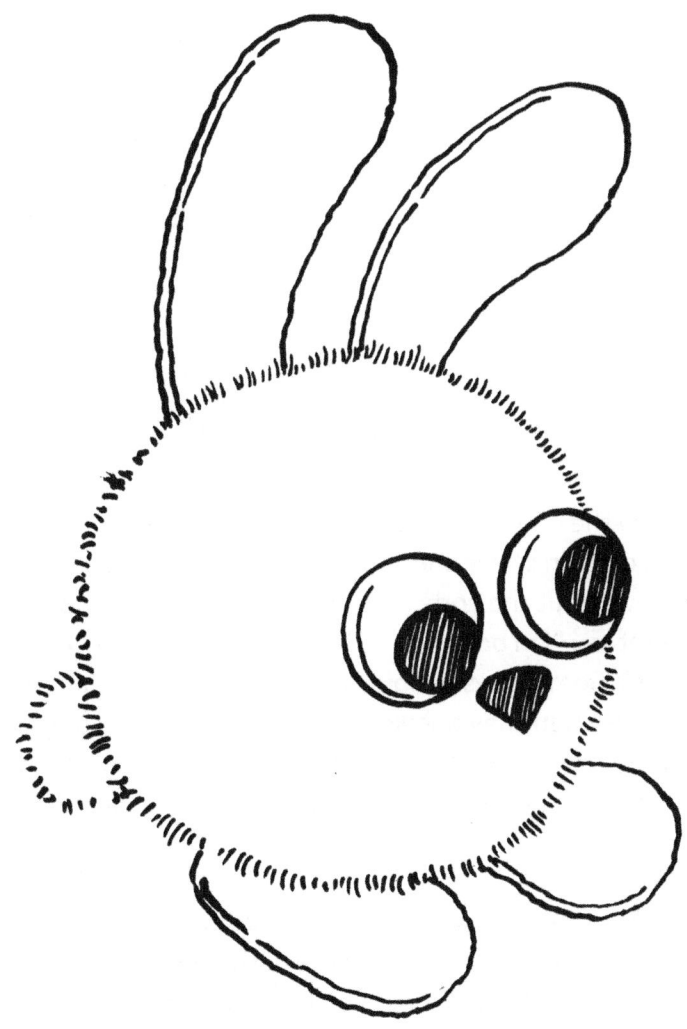

FIGURE 5.5 PET WORRY EXAMPLE

# Codes

This activity helps children and families explore the feelings of anxiety that may be underlying some of their behaviors.

## What you'll need
You'll only need paper and markers or a pen.

## Introducing this activity
You can start this activity by asking if the child has ever made a code. If the child has, you can ask about this; if not, you can explain that codes are a way of hiding a message. Suggest that you make a code together—you can create a simple code by allocating a figure for each letter in the alphabet. An example is provided below. You can then take it in turns to write something in the code and give it to each other to decipher.

## Example code

| | | | |
|---|---|---|---|
| 1 – A | 8 – H | 15 – O | 22 – V |
| 2 – B | 9 – I | 16 – P | 23 – W |
| 3 – C | 10 – J | 17 – Q | 24 – X |
| 4 – D | 11 – K | 18 – R | 25 – Y |
| 5 – E | 12 – L | 19 – S | 26 – Z |
| 6 – F | 13 – M | 20 – T | |
| 7 – G | 14 – N | 21 – U | |

Talk with the child about how the code serves to hide the message and how difficult it would be to understand the message if you didn't have the code. You can illustrate this point by trying to decode one of the child's messages without the code. Then you can talk about how people sometimes use code—for example, we might say "I'm bored" or "This is dumb" when we are worried that we might not be able to complete a task. Sometimes people hide their worried feelings underneath behaviors, such as avoiding other people when they are worried about what they might think or arguing and yelling with their parents about having to go to school. You can talk about other examples of children using code when they are anxious and wonder about whether the child also uses code.

## What families can do
Families can be included in the code activity, and parents may be able to provide their own examples of when they use code. If parents are not present for the activity, you can show them the codes later or give them a code to solve and explain how worried feelings can sometimes be hidden.

   This activity normalizes the experience of sometimes masking our worries. It is important to ensure that you present examples so that families realize that this pattern is common and do not perceive the child as being deceptive.

Talking with families about how they can better recognize code at home is helpful, as is talking with the child and parents about how they can find ways to share the underlying feeling rather than using code.

## Developmental considerations

Most mid-to-upper primary school children will be able to understand codes. Younger children or those with developmental difficulties may find this activity a little too demanding, both in terms of being able to make codes and relating this activity to how people manage their feelings. Their parents may, however, benefit from this activity, with a focus on learning to tune into the feelings under their child's behavior.

# Helpful vs unhelpful worry throw

This activity helps children identify helpful as opposed to unhelpful worries. This is useful in building their awareness of how anxiety works and how it can at times be useful.

## What you'll need

You will need some soft balls or beanbags and two large baskets or boxes. Some sticky notes or paper and Blu Tack® (poster putty) are often helpful for labeling the baskets or boxes. If the child prefers tabletop activities, rather than making this a throwing game, you can write each of the worries on a piece of paper and the child can sort them into paper bags.

## Introducing this activity

Talk with the child about how you have noticed that some of the worries they have are helpful and some are less helpful. Suggest that together you might be able to sort out which are which.

Set up the baskets or boxes, labeling one "helpful" and the other "unhelpful." Explain that having both helpful and unhelpful worries is usual and describe a situation in which you have had this experience. For example, you might recall feeling a little worried about a test when you were at school and studying hard because of this, which might have helped you to get good results. Being a little worried about big dogs you don't know is also helpful. An unhelpful worry, however, might be worrying so much about going on a high waterslide that you didn't try. Then describe a worry you might have and ask the child whether that would be helpful or unhelpful, encouraging them to throw it into the correct basket. Continue to name and throw worries that are helpful (those that helped you to stay focussed and work hard on something or helped keep you safe) into the helpful basket and throw unhelpful ones (those that led to you feeling worse or caused you to avoid the situation) into the unhelpful basket.

Work through other examples with the child, helping them to identify helpful and unhelpful worries. Starting with general ideas and moving toward examples that relate more to the child's experience is usually a good way to work. When asking about a worry, you can talk about whether it would be a little bit of a worry or a big one, as often children come to discover that little worries can be helpful while bigger ones can be unhelpful. For example, worrying a little about what others might think of you might be useful when you meet new people in that it might ensure that you are polite and remember to use your manners; on the other hand, worrying too much might mean you avoid meeting new people or don't talk when you do meet them.

## What families can do

If parents are in the session, they may be able to identify helpful and unhelpful worries of their own. If parents are not in the session, you can talk with them afterwards about the game and ask about any helpful or unhelpful worries they notice their child having. Talk together about what parents might be able to do when they notice unhelpful worries. Perhaps the child would be happy for their parents to comment without judgment on any unhelpful worries they notice (e.g., "I'm wondering if that worry is a helpful one or an unhelpful one...").

## Developmental considerations

Younger children and those with developmental difficulties may need support to understand the concept of helpful and unhelpful worries. This may still be an appropriate activity to use with these children and their parents, particularly with families where there is little ability to tolerate anxiety and parents don't want their children to experience any anxiety.

For children who have experienced trauma, there may be worries that have been helpful and kept them safe in the past but are no longer necessary. For example, worrying that disagreements will result in violence may have been protective at one point but is no longer relevant. Ensuring that children have had the opportunity to work through these experiences and that parents have understood these responses is, however, essential prior to using this framework and it is important to acknowledge the helpful role these worries once had.

# Worry cloud

This activity is useful for helping children to assess the impact of their worries and identify more helpful thoughts. It also incorporates a breathing strategy.

## What you'll need
You will need some cotton balls, some cardboard and some markers.

## Introducing this activity
Ask the child about what cloudy days are like. Can they see the sun? Why not? Where might the sun be? What would need to happen so they could see it?

Explain that sometimes worries are like clouds. They make everything seem dark and gray and stop us from seeing the light of the sun. Some days are cloudy, just like some days we have more worries. Importantly, clouds pass; they come and go, and so do worries. Suggest that you use some cotton balls to make a cloud. Using a marker, draw the outline of a cloud on the cardboard and place lots of cotton balls within the outline.

Give the child a simple example of a worry cloud. For example, you might talk about how you sometimes worry about being late and explain how this makes you feel angry or stressed. Then talk about how the worry cloud gets in the way of you seeing some important things. Suggest that you blow away the worry cloud together so that you can see some of the important things. Using big breaths in through the nose and out through the mouth, blow the cotton balls from the cloud and write or draw some of those important things inside the outline. For example, you might write "I'll only be a little late" or "Everyone runs late sometimes" or even "It will be ok," depending on the child you are working with and the complexity of thoughts that are appropriate to them.

Once the child has understood the concept, do this using a worry that relates to their experience and some helpful thoughts or important things to remember that are relevant to the child. You can talk about the way their body feels when they are worried, the sorts of thoughts they have when they are worried and what they notice about how they behave or act depending on where you are at in therapy. You can ask them to practice blowing away their worry cloud and remembering the helpful things that may have been hidden by it, reflecting on how they feel after doing so.

## What families can do
Parents can be engaged directly in this activity by getting them to think about their own worry clouds and having a go at blowing these away. Children can also take their worry clouds home and show them to other family members, demonstrating how they blow the worry clouds away. Parents can also be encouraged to continue to use this language at home—for example, by noticing those times when their child seems to only be able to see the worry clouds and wondering what they might see if they were to blow the worry clouds away.

## Developmental considerations
This activity can be used in a simplified format with younger children if you focus simply on having them blow the worry cloud away. Children with developmental difficulties may find it difficult to

associate clouds with worries and are likely to need some repetition to do so. Older children can engage in the more complex procedure described above in which they need to reflect on what else they could notice or how they might be able to challenge the worries (depending on the theoretical framework you are using).

# Tunnel vision worry

When children are worried, they tend to overestimate how likely it is that bad things will happen and how bad they will be. They also tend to underestimate their ability to cope if something does happen. This activity helps children and families to reflect on common thinking errors the child may be experiencing and helps them to think more realistically.

## What you'll need
You will need a cardboard tube from an empty roll of paper towel or similar, paper, markers, scissors and sticky tape or glue.

## Introducing this activity
Tell the child that you were thinking about what it means to have tunnel vision. Take it in turns to look through the cardboard tube and reflect on what you can see. Talk about what you might think if that was all you could see. For example, you might be able to say that, looking through the window with the tube, all you can see is a tree; and if you weren't able to look without the tube, you might not know that there are buildings and a road.

After playing for some time in this way, you can talk about having noticed that anxiety often gives us tunnel vision. Use some examples that are relevant to the child. For example, you might talk about how when they are worried about going to school they often think that something really bad will happen to their mom even though bad things rarely happen. Talk about how they might look through their worry tunnel and only see this outcome. To emphasize this point you can write it on some paper so that you can see it through the tunnel or stick it to the end of the tunnel so it is the only thing you can see when you look through.

Reflect on how anxiety might stop the child from seeing the bigger picture, and talk about what they might see or know if they weren't feeling anxious. For example, the child might talk about knowing that their mom makes good choices and this helps her to stay safe, or that really bad accidents are very rare. Together, write these things down and cut them out, leaving some space below the writing for a flap. Fold the paper then stick the flap to the top of the tube, so that the pieces of paper stand up and are easily seen, as shown in Figure 5.6. This adds to the experience of seeing the bigger picture when the child looks outside of the tunnel.

## What families can do
Parents can have a turn at looking through the worry tunnel and can reflect on how they would feel if all they could see was the worry. They may be able to think of examples in which anxiety has given their child tunnel vision. Parents may be able to normalize this experience by offering an example of a time that their own worry caused them to have tunnel vision.

Talk with parents about when they notice their child looking through the worry tunnel and discuss with the child ways in which parents might be able to help when they notice this. For example, the child may be happy for the parent to say, "I wonder if you are looking through your worry tunnel right now?" and "What would you see if you looked outside of the tunnel?"

## Developmental considerations

This activity is best for older children in mid-to-late primary school as it requires children to reflect on thoughts and the concept is likely to be too advanced for many early primary school children.

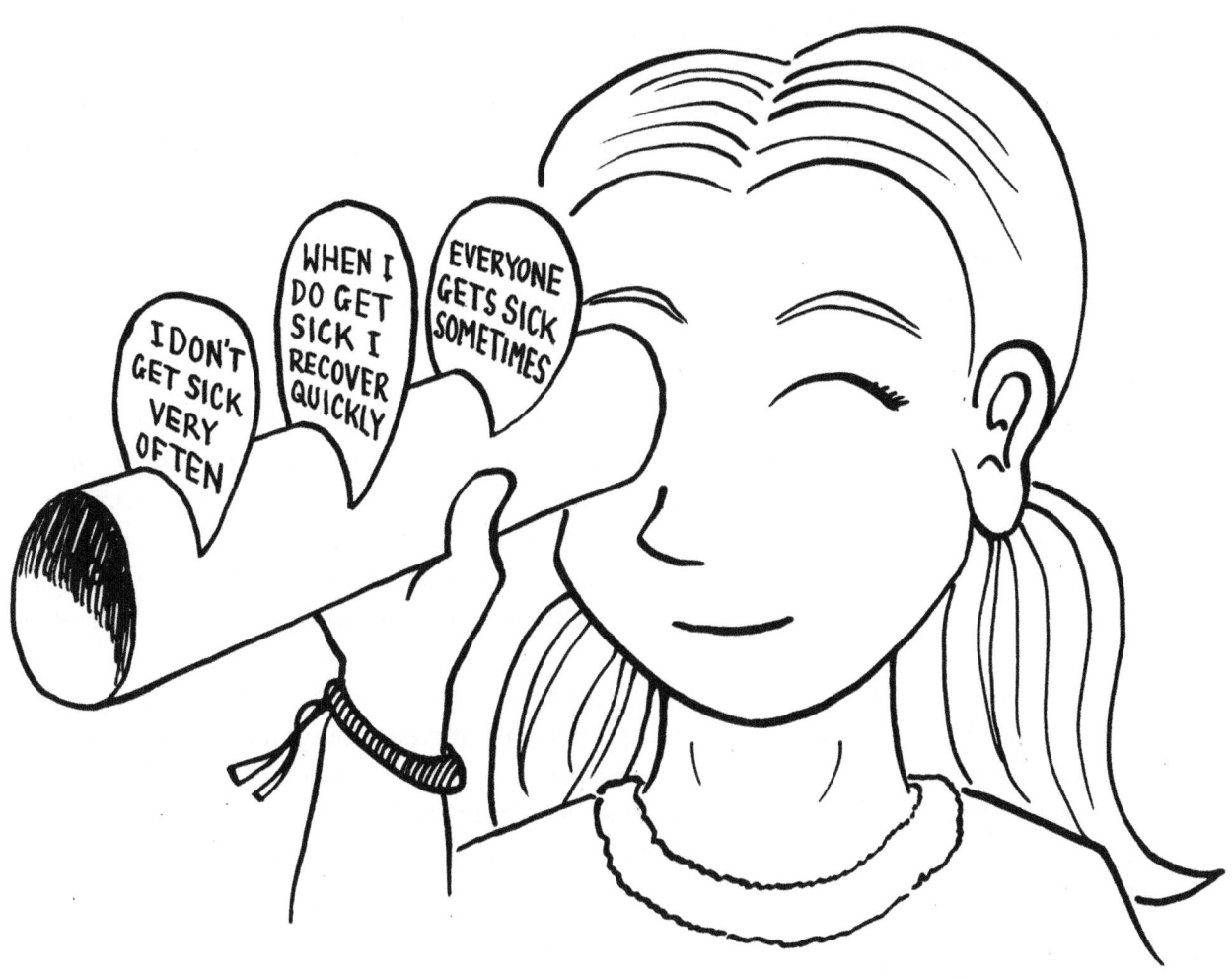

FIGURE 5.6 TUNNEL VISION WORRY EXAMPLE

# Another word for...

This activity assists in developing the emotional vocabulary children have and helps them begin to think about the strength of their feelings. It is particularly useful for children who tend to have big reactions and find it difficult to scale their feelings. For children who are anxious, being able to tune into lower levels of anxiety often places them in a better position to manage their worries. This activity also encourages the family to reflect on the language they use and how much they talk about feelings.

## What you'll need
You will need a large piece of paper to make a poster, and markers.

## Introducing this activity
Talk with the family about how you wonder about the words they use at home around feelings, and in particular around anxiety. For example, you might have heard them talk about feeling worried and wonder what other words they use at home that mean a similar thing. Suggest that some of these words might mean really, really, worried, such as terrified. Other words might just mean a little worried, such as concerned. Explain that having a good range of words helps us to measure the size of the feeling we are experiencing. Together, begin making a poster displaying all the similar words you can think of.

As the child and family generate words they use to describe anxiety, ask about how big that feeling is for them. Often, a useful way of scaling is to have children show you with their hands.

Depending on where you are at in therapy, you may also like to ask about how that anxiety feels in a child's body, what sort of thoughts they have and what they typically do in response to that feeling. Parents can also be engaged in conversation about how they respond when their child is feeling that way.

## What families can do
Families can complete this activity together; however, if this is not possible, then creating the poster in a session and sending it home for the family to add to is usually helpful.

Encouraging parents to check in with their child about their level of anxiety at home using some of the words on the poster is important. For example, if the child has identified that frightened is a bigger feeling than really worried, a parent might be able to talk with a child about something they are fearing and wonder if they are frightened or just really worried.

## Developmental considerations
Younger children are likely to need more support from parents and the therapist to identify words. Helping them to link words overtly with the size of the feeling is important. For example, you might say, "Annoyed is like a little bit angry. Show me with your hands how big annoyed is?" Older children may enjoy ranking the words according to the size of the feeling.

# When to worry throw

This is a helpful activity for encouraging children to focus on the here and now and is particularly helpful for children who tend to worry about the future.

## What you'll need
You will need some paper and some Blu Tack® (poster putty), along with some markers. You will also need a soft ball.

## Introducing this activity
Explain to the child that you have noticed that they often worry about things that have yet to occur. Say that you have been wondering when would be a good time to worry about these things and that you would like to play a game about this. Talk with the child about when they may worry about these events, and choose some time frames, writing one on each piece of paper. For example, you might write "now" on one piece of paper, "tomorrow" on another, "next week" on another and "next year" on another. Be guided by the language the child comes up with around time frames; however, try to have a reasonable range and remember that you can add additional time frames as you move through the activity. Blu Tack® each piece of paper to the wall and give the child a soft ball.

Provide the child with an example, such as whether or not to buy a house, and ask the child when would be a good time to worry about that. Have the child throw the ball at the time frame that they think is right. Using an example of something that is clearly an adult worry usually helps children to understand that this is not something they need to worry about anytime soon. Provide further examples and work up to using some of the child's worries.

Children will generally recognize that these things should be worried about far later, and you can often talk about if and when these things happen as being the right time to worry about them. Indeed, some children may like to add a piece of paper saying "when it happens." If, however, a child identifies that they should worry about this in the short term, you can talk about what it will be like worrying about that, along with numerous other worries. Talk about how exhausting that would be and wonder what it would be like to put some of those worries off until later.

## What families can do
Often, parents can get caught up in worrying about the future. For example, they might be worrying about whether their child might get into a good university, rather than focusing on enjoying primary school. Some parents will benefit from this activity themselves and if they are in the session, they might be able to identify some examples of their own. If parents are not in the session, they are likely to find hearing some common parent examples helpful. You can encourage them to watch out for when their child is worrying too far ahead and suggest that they take some of the time frame pages home and put them on the fridge so they can all remind each other about this.

## Developmental considerations
This activity requires that children have an awareness of their worried thoughts. Children also need to have a basic concept of time and to be able to identify which page refers to which time frame.

Younger children are likely to find this difficult. You can simplify the time frames somewhat by listing some ages (e.g., is this a "6-year-old worry," a "12-year-old worry," or a "20-year-old worry") and having the child identify what age they think will be a good age to begin worrying about that particular worry.

# CHAPTER 6

# BUILDING COPING SKILLS

Anxious children benefit from developing their coping skills. This includes calming their body and building their relaxation and problem-solving skills, and can be assisted by developing helpful narratives or stories about the anxiety as well as increasing a child's focus on their strengths and values. In this chapter we touch briefly on each of these areas and provide a number of therapeutic activities.

## Calming the body

### LULU

Lulu (9 years) had been in therapy for a few months. She would become anxious in response to a broad range of triggers and would respond in anger. Her parents were beginning to tune into early warning signs that she was becoming anxious, which was difficult as these were subtle and Lulu tended to escalate quickly. Lulu's mother arrived for one therapy session very excited. She'd been able to notice some of the early warning signs and gently approach her daughter, putting an arm around her shoulder and wondering if perhaps she was worried. Lulu had burst into tears and been able to talk about her worry in response to this.

Parents are essential in helping children learn to calm their bodies, which is necessary in learning to manage anxiety. Bruce Perry speaks about this process as needing to regulate, relate and reason. Perry's model has a basis in neuroscience and originates from his work on trauma (Perry and Dobson 2010). However, it is useful for all children and fosters the process of co-regulation. Regulation involves calming the child's body. For a toddler this means picking them up and holding them, whereas for an older child it might be about an arm around their shoulders, encouraging them to take a walk with you, or offering them a cold drink. Providing the body with other forms of sensory input often allows the child to regulate and calm and enables us to move onto relating. Relating involves the naming and empathizing we talked about in Chapter 5. Sometimes when this isn't working for parents it's because they are not regulating their child prior to relating to them. They are trying to relate and reason with children who are in a state of high anxiety and are unable to engage those thinking parts of their brain that would allow them to register what is being said. Relating involves naming and empathizing and sitting with the feeling prior to moving on to reasoning, which involves thinking about how the child can manage the situation.

For a younger child who is nervous about going somewhere new for the first time, a parent carrying them while kindly acknowledging that they are a little worried might be a good way to regulate and relate. The parent might then be able to move on to the reasoning stage, perhaps suggesting they read a book together or play in the sandpit. With an older child who is anxious before a concert and is unsure if they want to go onstage, a parent might regulate by giving them a squeeze, relate by sharing that they too always get nervous before performances, and reason by asking what might help.

If you have children, you may have observed how powerful this strategy can be. You may also have observed it in the clinic room. We often utilize this strategy when emotions come into the room, offering a child something that helps them to regulate themselves. This might involve using something sensory. For example, we have sequined cushions in our clinic rooms that children love to stroke and draw patterns on. It might involve connecting physically with a parent, getting a drink of water or even just having some time alone.

It is important to acknowledge that children with emotional difficulties can take a lot longer to regulate. For example, children with an autism spectrum disorder, those with a trauma background and even those who have limited experience with regulating their emotions can take much longer to calm their bodies. Helping children and families tune into and prioritize calming their bodies is a key aspect of therapy; if missed, it can impact on their ability to engage in further therapy. For example, a child who struggles to tune into and calm their body is unlikely to be able to use cognitive strategies they might learn in therapy.

The idea of regulating and relating prior to reasoning can be difficult for parents too. A parent might be encouraged to hug their child to regulate them in situations where they previously scolded them and this may seem counterintuitive. Often it helps to acknowledge this openly in therapy and provide a rationale for why this strategy works. For example, most parents can empathize with how hard it is to talk when they are anxious or angry and can appreciate that calming down might allow them to problem-solve more rationally. It often helps to explain that children are unable to use their thinking brain when they are very anxious, so in that state they can't think rationally, make considered choices, or learn from consequences. Modeling this strategy in sessions can also help parents to understand how valuable it can be.

Sometimes parents can struggle to calm their children before problem-solving because they are short on time or are faced with multiple demands, such as needing to soothe two children at once. At other times the situation can make it difficult to calm a child. Consider, for example, a child who is in the back seat of the car feeling very anxious and upset while you are driving on a freeway. It's important that as therapists we remain mindful of these challenges and accept that all parents will have times when it is difficult to calm their children or when they respond in ways that escalate rather than regulate their child. It is essential to ensure that parents feel able to talk openly with a therapist about this without feeling blamed.

## Breathing and relaxation

### JUAN

Juan was an 8-year-old with an autism spectrum disorder who often experienced some end-of-term fatigue, which resulted in increased anxiety and behavioral difficulties. His mother was able to notice the pattern early one term and she and the therapist engaged Juan in a discussion about what might help him to relax. His mother and therapist were able to talk about how he could choose to have some more time at home and he decided to have a week off from his extra-curricular activities. Juan enjoyed the downtime and was able to manage the end of term better than he had previously.

Breathing is a useful way of learning to calm your body; however, it does require practice in order for it to be useful (Hudson *et al.* 2019). When experiencing moments of anxiety, we tend to breathe faster and our breathing is shallower. Tuning into and being able to regulate our breathing is therefore very helpful.

Helping children to notice and modify their breathing is easier with older children. The younger the child, the more support and practice they are likely to need. A key aspect of teaching breathing is enabling the child to see the impact of their breath. The box below contains a number of ideas and activities for helping children to see their breath. The activity *Splattering worries* (page 129) can also be used to teach children about breathing.

---

### Useful ideas for helping children to see their breath

Blowing bubbles.

Blowing a windmill toy.

Blowing cotton balls across a table or off their hand.

Blowing through a straw into a glass of water and making bubbles.

Blowing paint across a page to create a breath painting.

Giving a child a toy to place on their stomach as they lie down and breathe.

Putting the child's hand on their stomach and noticing it move as they breathe.

Placing the child's hand in front of their mouth to notice their out-breath.

---

Ideally, children learn to slow their breathing and breathe deeply for a couple of minutes, focussing on having a long out-breath through their mouths. For many children, however, a couple of minutes is a long time to stay still and focus on something like breathing. Being realistic about your expectations is important; however, even if you feel it highly unlikely that the child would manage more than one deep breath, there is still value in promoting this. First, taking a single deep breath provides a pause, and for many children with anxiety pausing is something that can support them to choose a response rather than react with a flight, fight or freeze response. Second, a single deep breath emphasizes the value of breathing and tuning into your body and this may be something that children can extend on when they are older.

Practice is essential with breathing and this needs to be supported by the family. We would ask that a parent or someone else within the family make the commitment to practice breathing with the child if we are asking for a daily breathing practice. If we are working on a single deep breath, then we would also encourage parents to practice this. Children love to prompt their parents to breathe; if you have a parent who will engage in this in a playful manner, this is a good way of supporting the child to take breathing from the clinic room and formal practice into their day-to-day lives.

The other element that we need to keep in mind when teaching breathing is how readily this can be applied in the context of the child's life. Many of the ideas in the box above are useful for helping children see the impact of their breath; however, they are unlikely to generalize to their day-to-day life unless the therapist supports the child in making this extension. For example, in the *Splattering worries* activity (page 129) the therapist has the child practice pretending to blow the paint away, talking with them about how this is something they could do at school or at soccer, even though they won't really have paint with them.

In addition to breathing, some children will readily engage in other formal relaxation practices, such as visual imagery or progressive muscle relaxation, or they may be happy to engage in mindfulness practices. Again, we need to think about how these practices can be incorporated into the child's and family's daily routine in a regular and enjoyable way. In general, we find that children are more likely to engage if they can find recordings or apps that appeal to them and if the practices are kept brief (even just a few minutes). Practices that involve movement or sensory aspects also tend to be more engaging. That said, not all children will want to engage in formal relaxation or mindfulness practices, and not all families will be able to support this with regular practice. Given that children are naturally mindful and relaxed when they are playing, we can also think about play as an opportunity for mindfulness and relaxation practice.

It is helpful to think about relaxation more generally—for children this means thinking about play. Children today are more heavily scheduled than ever before. Time for unstructured play is very limited and the decrease in unstructured playtime has been associated with an increase in children's anxiety (Gray 2011). Clearly this data is correlational and there are likely to be a number of factors at play, but it is worth considering. Many playful activities that children enjoy have the effect of directly calming the body and can become a regulating strategy for them. Physical activities such as jumping on a trampoline, riding a bike, or free dancing are calming in the moment and helpful for managing anxiety in an ongoing way. Sensory and creative activities can also be calming for children (e.g., listening to music, playing with modeling clay, or drawing), as can time outside in nature.

Talking with the families you work with about the structure of their week, how they can avoid overscheduling and ensure that there is time for relaxation and unstructured play is important. There are many challenges for families in this regard. Some are cultural, with families feeling the need to enrol their children in a number of extra-curricular activities; and some are practical, with many families needing both parents to work. It is important to be mindful of these constraints when talking with families and help them to think about what is working for them and whether there is anything they can do to free up time in their week. Sometimes making even a small change can support the whole family to feel a little more relaxed. For example, one creative family I worked with shared cooking dinners with a neighbor, which freed them up to spend more time with their children in the afternoons.

Exploring with the child what they find relaxing is also important. For some children this might be shooting hoops outside, whereas for others it might be reading a book. Sometimes parents have not understood that the child finds this relaxing and they might feel frustrated by the amount of time their child spends engaged in what they view as an unproductive activity. Being able to clarify this in therapy and emphasize the importance of children doing things they enjoy is useful. Parents often benefit from tuning into what helps their child to relax. They may gain a better understanding of their child, find they get a bit more time to themselves or notice that their child is calmer as a result of relaxing more. When having this discussion, parents often begin thinking about their own relaxation strategies and this can be a useful way of talking about self-care with them.

## Problem-solving and resilience

### MY SON

My 9-year-old son is making muffins for breakfast as I'm writing this at the kitchen bench on a lazy holiday morning. I don't use a recipe when making muffins, so when he asks about how much milk or oil to add, my response is that he should add some and see how that goes. It's slightly uncomfortable for him as he loves raspberry muffins and would like them to turn out well; however, he is adding and adjusting, and the batter is looking good. As he is scooping the mixture into the tray (having confirmed that it tastes good), he looks proud of himself. I suspect his pride is greater than it would be if I had given him a recipe. He has also had another experience that has emphasized that it is ok to try and then try again if it's not quite right.

## CHIARA

Chiara was an anxious 12-year-old. She struggled to make decisions and felt anxious in social situations. The therapist engaged her in a number of hands-on activities that allowed her to try solutions and adjust them as needed. For example, when making a bath bomb with her therapist, she needed to add and adjust the amount of water and dry ingredients a number of times to get the mixture right. Chiara also had the experience of having one of the bath bombs fall out of the mold and she suggested that perhaps it could be bath salt instead. Her increasing ability to manage challenges in session paralleled her growing resilience in her day-to-day life.

Resilience involves being able to try something different if something doesn't work. It's about being able to adjust and respond and continue to try, knowing that we won't always get it right. Sometimes as therapists, however, we forget this when working with children. Many therapy programs teach children to problem-solve, with a view to identifying a more functional response to feared situations. Often in this context children are encouraged to stop and think about all their options and choose the best one, which implies that there is a right one.

From a developmental point of view this is challenging too. Weighing options is a cognitively difficult task that involves predicting outcomes, which is hard for younger children. Even for older children this requires significant cognitive abilities. More generally, problem-solving is a complex cognitive task that involves multiple skills, such as attention, working memory and cognitive flexibility.

Problem-solving is also time-consuming. If a child is in line to go on a flying fox (zip-wire) and is feeling anxious about this, the remaining children in the line are unlikely to take kindly to the child pausing and thinking for several minutes at the top of the line. Finally, choosing the best option implies that this option is likely to work, but that is not always the case. Sometimes even our tried-and-tested strategies don't work and we need to try something different. This is particularly important with children who are anxious. Having a solution not work can create further anxiety, so it is useful to promote the idea that the child can try something and see how that goes, then try something else if they need to.

It is important to clarify that pausing and thinking is something that we encourage. Rather than thinking about all of the options and choosing the best, we find thinking of one thing to try tends to be useful. The simplicity of this approach also works well for children who are anxious. When children are anxious, their ability to use their thinking brain and think logically is diminished, making it hard to think of a range of options. *Moves for life* (page 157) is helpful for exploring the value of pausing and thinking before acting.

Craft activities provide a great vehicle for exploring this problem-solving approach, as noted above with Chiara. There are a number of activities in this book that focus more directly on encouraging children to pause and use their thinking brain and develop their problem-solving skills using the approach above. These include *Jumping ponds* (page 131) and *Maze changes* (page 137).

Problem-solving is a pro-social skill that is often a focus in therapy. There are times, however, when it becomes clear in the therapy process that a child lacks other essential social skills and that this may be contributing to the anxiety they experience. If this is the sort of work you are able to do in therapy, then spending some time on this is likely to be valuable. Otherwise, referring the child to an appropriate social skills group is often the best option.

More generally, it is important that we support families to think about how their child can have experiences that build resilience and problem-solving skills. As noted earlier, children spend less time engaged in unstructured play now, the essence of which is arguably about exploring and experimenting. In play, children take risks and try out new behaviors. Sometimes they assess physical risk, such as knowing how high they can climb up a tree, and at other times they assess social risk, like knowing how much they can dominate the game before others get annoyed. They try out different ways of responding. For example, an anxious child who avoids social situations might play with their dolls, enacting more socially extroverted behavior. Play provides children with the opportunity to make mistakes and try out different options if one doesn't work. Cooperative play involves many social skills, with children negotiating and planning together. All of these aspects are likely to promote resilience and therefore reduce anxiety and might explain part of the relationship noted earlier between children having less unstructured play and being more anxious. It is essential therefore that we help families to think about how they can provide opportunities for play and experimentation. For many parents there can be a discomfort around messy play or around play that does not involve close adult supervision, so exploring this is essential.

A related point is that when children do more they feel more able to take on new challenges. Helping parents understand the value in having their child take on household chores and be developing new skills is important. For anxious children this might mean consciously thinking about what else they can be adding to this, such as beginning to go out to the letterbox alone and collect the mail. The sense of achievement that comes from learning to do new things and gradually becoming more independent is marked and can help an anxious child begin to think differently about their capacity to face new challenges.

## Externalizing, storytelling and other narrative therapy ideas

### IRIS

Iris was an 11-year-old girl nearing the end of therapy for anxiety. A younger family friend had been experiencing some anxiety and Iris had been sending her short videos with ideas about how she could manage this. In addition to being very helpful for her friend, these videos reinforced Iris's sense of achievement and reminded her of all of the strategies she had used to manage her own anxiety.

Narrative therapy works well for anxiety issues and is generally a good fit for children. It involves the use of language to distance and externalize the problem from the person. For anxious children this usually involves naming the worry. Naming the worry and talking about it as though it is external to the child has some clear advantages in that the worry becomes the problem rather than the problem being located within the child. It often unites parents and children in their desire to beat the worry and empowers the child, who begins to see the worry as "other." The narrative approach of externalizing lends itself to a playful approach. Children may come up with a name for their worry, such as Mr. Worry Pants or Worrywart, and can often be readily engaged in a "quest" or an "epic battle" against the worry. The box below includes some useful narrative questions to use with children and families. "The worry" can be substituted for whatever name the child chooses.

---

### Questions that help children externalize their worry

What does [the worry] make you do?

What is it like when [the worry] is around?

What is it like when [the worry] is not around?

What does [the worry] say to you?

How does your body feel when [the worry] is around?

Are there times when you manage to beat [the worry] even just a little?

What would you say to [the worry] if you met it in the street?

How old do you feel when [the worry] does that?

---

Most children will happily engage in these narrative conversations, which can be used right from your first session with the child. Parents can also find this way of talking about the worry very helpful. Some parents may need an explanation about why it is helpful to talk about the worry in this manner, though something like "I find that naming the worry makes it easier for us to talk about it" is usually sufficient. Occasionally I have had children who resist engaging in narrative conversations around their worry. They have tended to be older children who have been worried for a long period of time, and the worry appears to have become so intertwined with their sense of self that they find the conversation threatening. In this situation it is useful to move to an alternative approach, though you may be able to return to using a narrative approach later in therapy.

While externalizing is the most well-known of the narrative techniques, narrative therapy has far more to offer. One important aspect of narrative therapy is that it helps us to think about the stories we have, including the stories we have about our children. For example, a parent might have a story about their child that involves them being nervous and needing extra support. Often this narrative shapes the way the parent interacts with the child and so these stories have the potential to be self-fulfilling prophecies. From a narrative perspective we think about the need to thicken a story—that is, to weave in different elements and aspects, to make it more complex and less narrow. For example, noticing times that a child has been brave is a way of thickening a parent's narrative about their child. Gently noticing examples of this in session and also in the stories children and families tell us helps to highlight these aspects. Similarly, children who are anxious often have their own narratives that are about themselves not being able to cope or manage. Listening and noticing so that you can provide exceptions is an important intervention.

In addition, narrative therapy involves storytelling, an aspect that is readily integrated into play. For example, role play or puppet play that involves a story about worry can be very powerful for an anxious child. *Wise owl* (page 142) is a narrative puppet play activity. In play we can provide the child with alternative endings and in doing so open up possibilities. The child can observe and experiment with different ways of responding when anxious.

Creating stories is another useful intervention in therapy. Children who are reluctant to talk about their own worries can often be engaged in storytelling and will often share their worries in that context. For example, you can ask a child to tell you about the sorts of things children her age worry about, or you can have them create a story with you about an animal or character who has worries. Often this third-person approach provides children with some distance and gives them the freedom to express their experiences. Indeed, some children will prefer to work this way throughout therapy. Provided this work occurs in conjunction with changes in the child's day-to-day life, this is not a concern.

Another important aspect of narrative therapy involves witnessing a child's achievements. For example, certificates are a great way of acknowledging their progress. These can be shown to other family members or stuck to the fridge for visitors to see. The conversations that occur around certificates are a lovely way of thickening the narrative about a child's worries in addition to engaging the child's family system in the therapy process. Using narrative activities to highlight and share what the child has learnt is a great idea. For example, you can ask a child to tell you about the sort of things children her age worry about, or you can have the child create a story with you about an animal or character who has worries. They might even like to write a picture story book for younger children. *Expert news report* (page 144) is an activity that utilizes this strategy. In my practice we have created a folder of "Ideas for kids" where children can add a page with their own suggestions or reflections. It is kept in the waiting room and children love the experience of being asked to contribute to this.

## Focusing on what works and using strengths and values

### AMELIE

Amelie (6 years) frequently retraced her steps when leaving the house, becoming very upset and angry if her parents tried to hurry her or prevent this. She also engaged in a number of verbal rituals, insisting that her parents say "Yes, that's right" in response to questions that she asked. Amelie insisted on other routines within her day, such as her parents greeting her in a particular way and arranging her toys in her room in a particular manner. Her parents were able to identify that distraction often helped and noticed that Amelie engaged in fewer rituals when she did not attend after-school activities and had more time at home. Playing at home with her toys and her younger sister was important to Amelie and the therapist was able to focus on how her rituals could be reduced to allow for greater playtime.

Children benefit from learning a range of coping strategies for managing anxiety and often need support to bring together the strategies that they use. Feeling anxious can be overwhelming, so having a visual reminder of strategies makes them accessible and allows children and their parents to reference these as needed. In our book *Creative Ways to Help Children Manage Big Feelings* (Zandt and Barrett 2017) we provide several activities than can be used to highlight and consolidate a child's coping skills. *Putting it all together* (page 155) is another activity that supports children and parents to reflect on what has been helpful in managing their anxiety and to use those strategies more often.

We have already discussed a number of different coping strategies, but thinking more broadly about this can be useful. Children will often have some coping strategies that they have been using prior to coming into therapy and these can be included amongst their helpful strategies. For example, a child might love reading and find this to be a good coping strategy. The box below outlines the sort of strategies that can be useful to consider. When we are finishing up in therapy, reviewing these is even more important. Knowing what helped can be useful in managing future worries and may prevent relapse. In the short term, however, it also allows families to leave therapy feeling confident that they have the skills to manage future challenges.

---

**Coping strategies for children**

Playing with toys.

Reading or listening to stories.

Coloring, drawing or craft.

Physical activity (e.g., trampoline, ball play, bike riding, dancing).

Listening to or playing music.

Sensory toys.

Talking to a caring adult.

Patting a pet.

Nature or outside play.

Playing with siblings or friends.

Relaxation imagery.

Muscle relaxation (e.g., pretend to be a robot and then pretend to be a jellyfish).

Mindfulness practices.

Stretching.

Breathing techniques.

Helpful self-talk.

Using strengths and values is important when working with anxious children and their families. Children and families are often so depleted by the time they come in for therapy. Parents are focussed on the child's struggles and forget the child's strengths. Children who are struggling with anxiety feel unable to cope with the demands of their day-to-day lives and often their self-esteem suffers. All children have strengths and it is important that as therapists we uncover these and support children to utilize them, helping the children to shine. Parents and families have strengths too, many of which have been forgotten. Similarly, parents are often so busy just coping that they have lost sight of the bigger picture and what is important to them. Drawing out values in therapy can support a family to feel engaged and motivated and can map out the work that you do together.

Noticing strengths right from that first session can be really valuable. It provides a re-frame for the family and helps them to feel more empowered. Some of the strengths that you notice in the first session may indeed be some of the key strengths of the child and family and might be attributes that you utilize throughout therapy. Other times, however, a child and family's strengths will become more apparent as therapy progresses. Continuing to look for strengths throughout therapy is helpful, as is thinking broadly about strengths (e.g., interests, relationships, resources, personality traits, behaviors, strategies, and things they feel good about, enjoy or treasure). The activities *Shield ball* (page 149) and *Compliments box* (page 152) are helpful for exploring and highlighting a child's strengths.

ACT promotes the use of values in therapy and this is something that we find useful in our practice. It is important to remember that children are still developing their values and are likely to find it difficult to talk about the concept of values, which is quite abstract. Talking with children about what is important to them is often helpful, and older children will sometimes be able to engage in the discussion at this broad level. For younger children, however, values work often needs to be more specific and related to the difficulties they are identifying. For example, with a child who is socially anxious and desperately wants friends, you might be able to talk about what sort of friend they would like to be. Making that practical is essential. For example, if the child talks about wanting to be a kind friend, you might be able to consider what that involves, which might include saying hello. This would then give you a practical place to start and some direction for the therapy. Some of the activities in this book aim to help children focus on what is important to them. These include *My treasures* (page 146) and *Kicking toward my goal* (page 154).

Values are important to focus on with parents too. Sometimes parents get caught up in the specifics, and thinking about what they value is a good way to bring them back to the bigger picture. Asking about what they most want for their children or hearing about the key message they want to convey to their child is really valuable. Parents might feel that they want their children to be ok even when faced with challenges. Talking with them about what that would look like and what their child would need to do in order to achieve this can lead to the development of some shared goals. It can also support parents to evaluate how they are relating to their child currently and whether this is the most helpful approach both in the short term and the longer term. It provides a context to what you might be asking the parent to do and helps to align the therapeutic goals, giving both the parents and the therapist a clear aim.

# Holding on and breathing

This activity encourages children to explore what is meaningful and important to them, and supports them to pause and hold onto this when they are anxious.

## What you'll need

You will need paint and a selection of stones—preferably flat ones in a range of sizes. It is important to choose stones with a porous surface, rather than a glossy finish, as this will allow them to be painted.

Some children will prefer to have something that is soft and squishy, so having some stress balls as an alternative to the stones is useful. It is helpful to have a range of stress balls in different colors and shapes that the child can choose from. Colored permanent markers can be used to decorate the stress balls and can also be used as an alternative to paint for the stones.

## Introducing this activity

Explain to the child that sometimes when we get anxious it can be hard to remember to pause and breathe. Suggest that it might be useful to have something they could hold onto that might remind them to do this.

Offer the child a stone and a stress ball and allow them to feel each one. Having the child describe how each one feels is a good way to ground them. Allow the child to choose whichever they prefer and encourage them to hold it while they take a breath.

Explain that sometimes when we are worried it is difficult for us to hold onto what is important to us. Provide an example that helps the child to understand this. For example, you might say that when you have a difficult day it is hard for you to remember how much your family loves you. Ask the child if they have ever had this experience and suggest that they might like to decorate the stone or the ball with those things that are important to them.

Stones can be decorated with markers or paint depending on the child's preference. Stress balls are best decorated with permanent markers. You may like to make your own stone or stress ball in the session to enable the child to see what you mean. Explain what you are doing as you are decorating. For example, you might draw a picture of some leaves and explain that you love hiking in the countryside.

Talk with the child about the things that are important to them, and how holding on or keeping in mind these things can be helpful when they are anxious. For example, thinking of a book they can read when they get home might be useful for an anxious child who doesn't want to go to school and loves reading.

Talk with the child about when they would most need the stone or stress ball. Wonder about how they would know they needed to pause and breathe. Try having a go at holding on and breathing in the session.

## What families can do

Family members can also create their own stones or stress balls and reflect on what is important to them. If they join in at the end at the session and there isn't time for them to complete their own, they may be able to reflect on what they would put on one if they were to make one.

Parents often benefit from hearing about what is important to their child. It is also helpful to talk with the child and parents together about how the parents would notice that their child needed their stone or stress ball, and how they might gently remind the child to hold on and breathe.

## Developmental considerations

Younger children would benefit from having parents in the session while you complete this activity to assist the child with examples of things they enjoy and care about, and so that you are able to talk to the parents about the value in pausing, breathing, and focusing on what's important to us. Younger children will also need modeling and prompting from parents to remember this when they are feeling anxious. Similarly, children with developmental difficulties are likely to benefit from these modifications.

Older children are better able to consider what is important to them, and to learn to use this strategy themselves. It is important to remember that, even for older children, values are constantly changing and developing.

Of course, it is important to ensure that children are safe. If a child has a history of throwing items when they are angry, then this activity would be best completed with a soft stress ball.

# Splattering worries

Breathing is a useful calming strategy for children. It supports them to regulate their bodies and take a pause; however, it can be difficult to teach. Young children need to see the impact of their breath when they are learning breathing, and all children can benefit from some visual imagery around their worries changing.

## What you'll need

You will need some paint and paper for this activity. Thinner paint works best as children can usually spread a blob of paint with their breath. Straws are also often useful for this activity as they help the child to direct their breath.

## Introducing this activity

Talk with the child about how when we worry we tend to breathe faster. Say that slowing down our breath helps our bodies to calm down and means that we can think more clearly.

Suggest that you use some paint to experiment with this. Blob some colored paint onto the paper to represent each worry. For example, you might take a turn first, saying that you sometimes worry about being late. You can then talk about how big a worry that is and match the size of the blob to the size of the worry. Children may also like to choose different colors for different-sized worries.

When you have some blobs on the paper, pause and notice what they look like. This is a good opportunity to talk about how your body might feel or the sorts of thoughts you might have when you experience those worries.

Suggest that you see what might happen if you blow the worries away. Show the child how to take a deep breath in through their nose and out through their mouth. Encourage the child to blow on the paper and see what happens. Blowing through a straw is often easier—at least to start with. Notice any changes in the child's body as they breathe too.

Some children may also like to talk about how the worries have changed. Perhaps they have moved or have become thinner and easier to see through. Or maybe they have mixed with other colors and become something different.

It is helpful to talk with the child about how they could blow their worries away when they are at school, home or other places relevant to the child. Together with the child, practice just pretending to blow the paint away. Talk with them about how they could do this and blow away their worries, even though they won't have paint with them.

## What families can do

Providing an explanation of the activity to parents is important to enable them to talk with their child about the ideas at home. If you have family members joining you at the end of a session, you could have the parents blow a worry and ask the child to explain what you have talked about. If you are sending the picture home for a child to show their parents, you might like to use a pen or marker to label each of the worries the child has blown so that they are able to see what the child named as worries.

## Developmental considerations

Younger children are likely to need their parents in the room when they talk about worries as they may find it difficult to name their concerns. You may also need to focus in on one aspect with younger children, such as how blowing through the straw makes their body feel. Children with developmental difficulties are likely to benefit from similar modifications. Older children, however, are usually able to engage in various aspects of the discussion around worries.

# Jumping ponds

Many anxious children worry about making decisions. Learning to problem-solve can be very challenging in this regard, with many models encouraging children to weigh up all of the possible options and choose the best one. Often children lack the ability to carefully consider options or they don't have the necessary time to do so. This activity emphasizes an alternative approach to problem-solving in which the child is encouraged to pause and think of something to try, see if it works and try something else if need be.

## What you'll need

You will need cardboard, scissors and markers. You might like to print the *Frog template* below onto green cardboard, or you can draw the frog freehand. You can use several small boxes as ponds or you can cut out cardboard ponds.

## Introducing this activity

Tell the child that you've noticed how hard it can be for them to make a decision at times and how this is something lots of people find difficult. Suggest that you make something to help you think about how to do this.

Draw a frog onto green cardboard or use the template to print. Encourage the child to cut it out and decorate as they wish. Suggest that together you make a home for the frog and also make some ponds out of boxes and/or cardboard. The key thing here is to ensure that the ponds are different shapes and sizes. It's useful to make at least three different ponds.

Ask the child which pond looks right for the frog and encourage them to put the frog in that particular pond. When the child does so, ask about how the frog feels in that pond. How does the frog's body feel? What would be a feeling word for that? If the frog is uncomfortable, suggest that the child have the frog take a breath, pause and then think about a different pond to try. You can repeat this process a few times.

Talk with the child about how sometimes it is like this for us. When we try something, we can tune into how we are feeling and can pause and breathe and decide if we need to try something different. You can link this in with examples from the child's life. Encourage the child to think about a decision they face and use the ponds to playfully explore their options.

Some children will like to pretend they are frogs and are jumping from one pond to another. Floor cushions make good ponds as they can be positioned on the floor so that the child can jump from one to another.

## What families can do

It is helpful for parents to understand the approach to problem-solving that you are encouraging with this activity and why this is likely to be helpful for the child. Having parents join in the activity or showing them how it was used can assist with this. Parents can prompt this approach at home when the child is faced with a problem, encouraging their child to pause, take a breath, and think of an option to try; then if it doesn't work out, repeating this process.

## Developmental considerations

This activity is great for younger and older children. Younger children will benefit from having a parent involved to assist in session and in continuing to model this approach to decision-making and problem-solving at home. Children with developmental difficulties can find it difficult to generate a range of options so may find this activity easier if they have a list of possible choices.

# Frog template

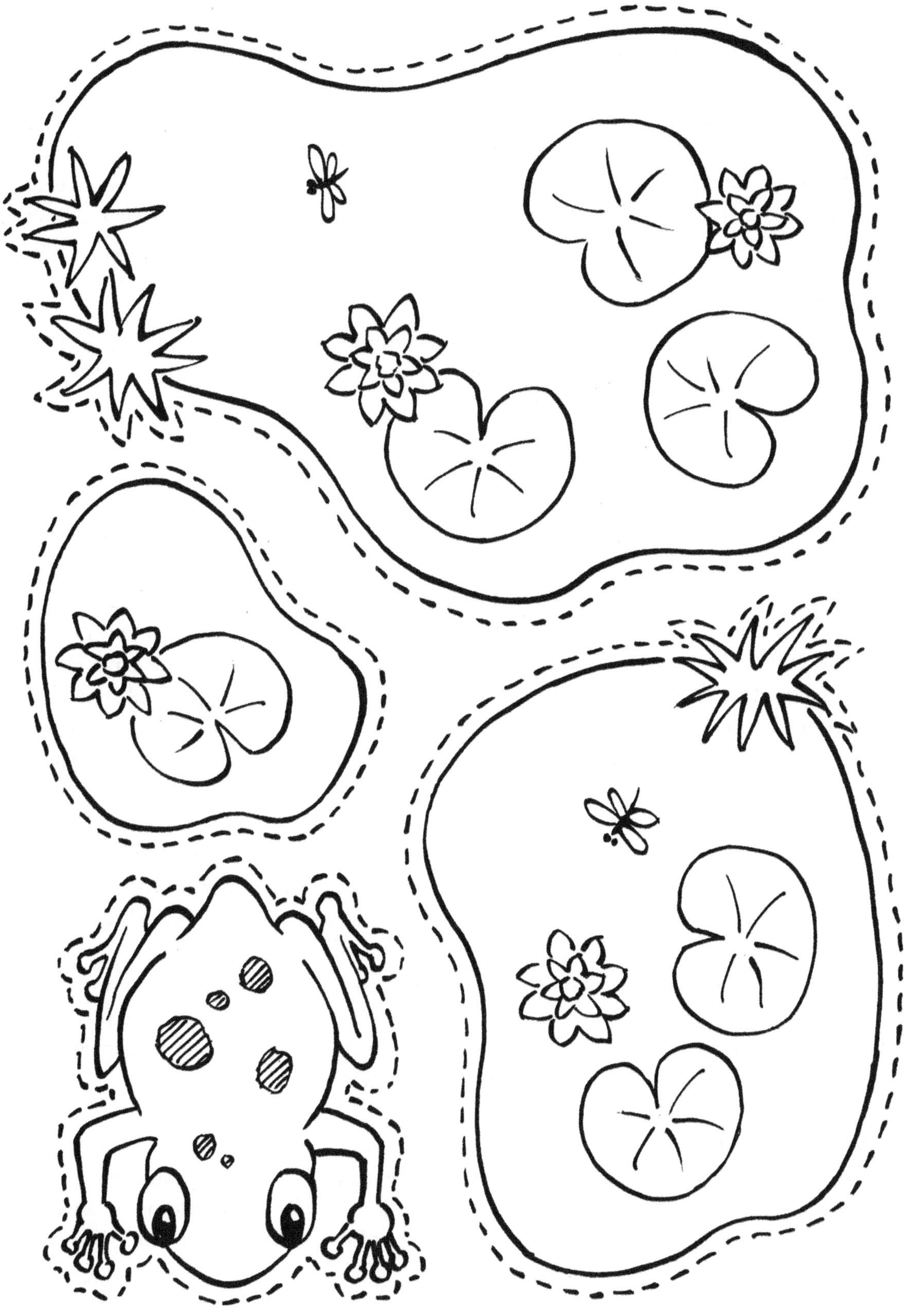

# Hitting the pause button

This activity helps children and families to recognize the role of pausing when feeling anxious, which provides an opportunity to regulate emotions and decide how to respond rather than simply react. Often children who are anxious will respond by avoiding the situation or becoming angry. Learning to notice their feelings and pause so they can use their thinking brain often supports children to make better choices and to negotiate situations they may otherwise have been unable to. It relies on children having a simple understanding of their thinking and feeling brain, so if you have yet to cover this it might be useful to look at the *Feeling and thinking brain* (page 100) activity first.

## What you'll need

You will need markers and a piece of cardboard, a craft foam sheet or a large popsicle stick to serve as your remote control. You may need scissors to cut your cardboard or foam to size. You might also like to use our *Remote control template* below.

## Introducing this activity

Remind the child that different parts of our brains have different and important jobs. Our feeling brain controls our feelings, helping us to react quickly to keep us safe when in danger, whereas our thinking brains can help us to use our memories and planning skills to decide how we want to respond. In order to turn our thinking brains on, we need to pause and calm our bodies.

Ask the child if they know what it means to pause, and talk about times when they have paused. Do they pause videos they are watching online or use the remote control to pause live TV? Suggest you make a remote control so you can practice some pausing. You can make a simple remote control using cardboard, craft foam or a large popsicle stick. The child can add whatever buttons they choose, though a pause button is the most important. If you like, you can use the *Remote control template*, coloring it then pasting it onto cardboard or foam.

When you have made the remote control, engage the child in some puppet play or role play and try using the pause function on the remote control to assist when the puppet or character is feeling anxious. For example, you might allow the child to be in charge of the remote control and enact some situations in which a puppet becomes worried and is unable to use their thinking brain. Encourage the child to choose when to push the pause button.

You can pair this with discussion about when the child knows they are beginning to become anxious and what helps them to pause. It's also good to reflect on what they can do that helps them to calm their body, with the understanding that this can turn on their thinking brain. For example, encouraging children to pause and take a deep breath is often helpful.

## What families can do

Parents can easily be involved in this activity. The child may be able to practice using the pause button on them and other family members in the session and at home, noting what it is about their facial expressions, body language and behavior that have led them to think it is a good time to pause.

If you don't have parents in the room when completing this activity, you can provide an explanation of what was covered in the session and ask the child to take the remote control home. This provides parents with a non-confrontational and fun way of assisting their child to better manage their feelings. Parents can allocate the remote control to one family member each day at home, encouraging them to be responsible for watching the other family members and letting them know if they need to pause.

## Developmental considerations

Many younger children will be able to benefit from this activity, particularly if you keep the language simple and practice in session as well as at home. Similarly, children with developmental difficulties often engage well in this activity when it is supported by practice at home. Older children still tend to enjoy this and may also be keen to think about other remote control functions, such as the rewind button.

# Remote control template

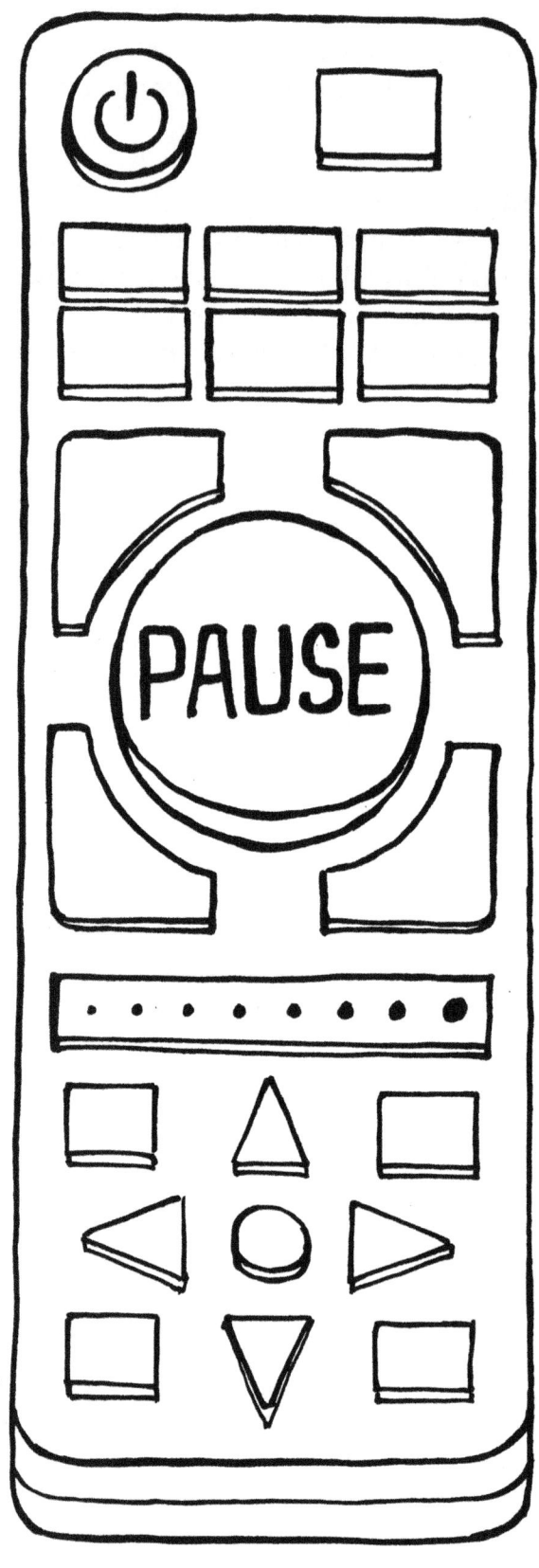

# Maze changes

This activity encourages children to feel comfortable making a different choice if something isn't going right. It helps them to discover that it's ok to try something different and encourages them to pause.

## What you'll need
You will need cardboard and either some wool/yarn or some matchsticks, as well as some craft glue.

## Introducing this activity
Wonder about whether the child has ever completed a maze and talk about what that was like. Suggest that you make one together and identify where the start and the end will be. You can then begin creating the borders of the maze, doing so by gluing the matchsticks or wool onto the cardboard. Some children will prefer to draw the maze outline prior to gluing the matchsticks or wool. Try to ensure that the borders of the maze are wide enough to run a finger through and try to include some dead-ends or wrong turns. You may like to make a maze at the same time as the child, particularly if you are working with a younger child who is likely to find the planning component of this tricky.

When the maze has been completed, ask if you can have a turn. Run your finger through the maze, reflecting as you do so at any decision points. For example, you might say, "I could go this way, but what if that is wrong—I'm worried it won't be right." Model that you can breathe and pause, thinking before you decide which way to go. Try to reflect on those times where you may make mistakes. For example, you might say something like "Oh, that isn't right. Next time I'll know not to go this way," taking a deep breath as you go back. Notice when you get to the end that even though it took you a long time, you did manage to get there. Encourage the child to have a go and help them to breathe and pause when they are faced with a decision point or have made a mistake.

After you've had a play, talk with the child about the sorts of decisions they are faced with in their life. Wonder about whether they breathe and pause before deciding, or indeed whether they spend so long deciding and worrying about making the wrong decision that they don't have a go. You may like to have them notice one thing that would be helpful when they have a decision to make and write this on the back of the maze for them to take home.

## What families can do
Allowing children to make mistakes is essential for their development and it can be something that parents of anxious children avoid. The maze is a good way to begin having a discussion about this and helping parents to provide their child with the space to develop their own problem-solving skills. For example, using the maze as a metaphor, parents can say something like "I can see you've got an idea. Why don't you try it. If it doesn't work you can always try something else."

Having parents in the session may provide an opportunity for noticing those times when they are tempted to jump in and prevent their child from making mistakes. This can allow for some helpful conversation. Alternatively, showing a parent the maze afterwards and having the child demonstrate some of the mistakes they made and how these impacted on their learning should help. Playing with the maze at home is a fun way to help reinforce these discussions.

## Developmental considerations

As noted above, younger children can struggle to plan out and make a maze. Having some printed onto cardboard so that they can simply glue the matchsticks or wool over the top can help. For those children who are likely to find gluing matchsticks too difficult because of their fine motor skills, popsicle sticks can be a good alternative. Similar modifications may be useful for children with developmental difficulties.

Older children who find mazes simple can complete this activity with their eyes closed, using the raised boundaries to guide their decision-making.

# The amazing time-traveling thinking brain

This activity helps children to think about their past experiences and likely outcomes when deciding what to do. Looking to the past is a way of looking for evidence, which is a key component of a CBT approach. Looking to the future promotes problem-solving and reinforces the need to pause and think when worried, encouraging children to decide rather than react. If you have yet to introduce the concept of the thinking and feeling brain to the child, then you should consider completing the *Feeling and thinking brain* (page 100) activity first.

## What you'll need
You will need a piece of wool or string, cardboard and markers or a pen. You might like to use the *Time-traveling brain template* below.

## Introducing this activity
Comment on how you've noticed that the child is pausing and using their thinking brain, and provide an example of this based on what the child or their parents have shared with you.

Explain that the thinking part of our brain is very powerful and can even time-travel, letting us think about how something has worked in the past and have a guess at how something might work in the future. Suggest that you make something so you can figure out how this works. Print and cut out the time-traveling brain templates or draw your own on cardboard. Punch holes in each of the pieces and thread them onto a piece of wool in the following order: the past, thinking brain, the future. Extend the piece of wool between your arms with the brain in the middle and the past and future on either side.

Provide the child with an example. For example, you might say that you were recently worried about swimming in the ocean. Move the brain back along the wool to the past while you explain how your thinking brain time-traveled back and you remembered that last time you were safe in the waves and had lots of fun. Then, move the brain along the wool to the future as you explain that you also thought for a minute and realized that you would be swimming in a patrolled area so that if anything happened you would be able to get help.

Provide some additional examples until the child understands the concept, then ask the child if they can think of a time when their thinking brain has time-traveled. Next, think of a situation they are worried about and move the brain along the wool exploring what might happen if they use their thinking brain to look at what has happened in the past or guess at what might happen in the future.

When presenting this to children it is useful to avoid getting too hooked into what might happen in the future. Promoting this as guessing and treating it lightly allows you to have a flexible approach to problem-solving, encouraging the child to try something different if things don't work out as they predicted. This is consistent with our approach to problem-solving more generally.

## What families can do
If families are in the session, they may like to provide examples of times that they have been able to have their thinking brains time-travel and think about the past or guess about the future. Showing

a family the time-traveling model at the end of the session and having the child explain as they move the brain along the wool is also a good way to involve families.

It is useful for parents to understand the way you are encouraging the child to consider the evidence from past experiences and to problem-solve by pausing and having a guess about the future. They can continue to use the metaphor of the time-traveling brain to reinforce these ideas at home, and the child can keep the time-traveling brain model to assist with this.

## Developmental considerations

This activity includes some more complex concepts and is likely to be best suited to mid-to-late primary school students. Similarly, you may need to keep this simpler with children with developmental difficulties, focussing on the brain traveling to either the past or the future until they are more readily able to integrate both.

# Time-traveling brain template

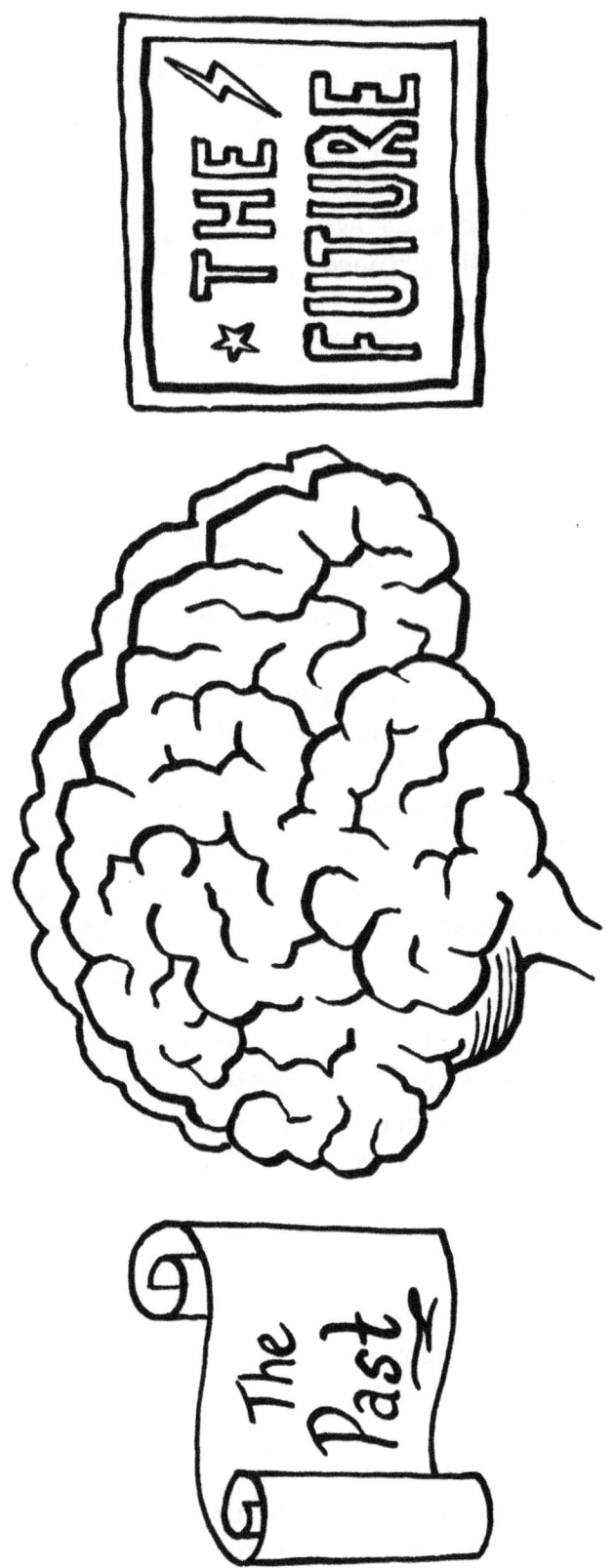

# Wise owl

This is a useful activity for helping children to consolidate coping strategies and improve their ability to generate helpful thoughts.

## What you'll need

You may like to print the *Owl template* below onto some light card, or you could have the child draw an owl onto the cardboard. You will also need a popsicle stick and some glue. Googly craft eyes are fun to add if you have them.

Alternatively, you can use an owl puppet if you have one in your collection. Having some other animal puppets or toys is also helpful.

## Introducing this activity

Explain to the child that you have some animals who need help with some of their worries. Suggest that the child be the owl puppet and that some of the animals might come and visit them for advice. Remind the child how wise owls are and that you know they will have lots of good ideas to help.

If you are making an owl, cut out the shape and stick it on the popsicle stick. Add googly craft eyes and decorate as the child desires.

If you have other puppets or toy animals available, choose a puppet or animal and act out a scenario with them. For example, you could be a little pig who is too scared to jump in the deep mud, or a horse who won't say neigh to the other horses because he thinks they won't like him. After providing a bit of an explanation of the character, suggest the animal goes to see the wise owl. Have your animal explain the situation to the wise owl and ask for the wise owl's advice.

Encourage the child to be the wise owl and see what they suggest to the other animal. If necessary, you can prompt the child for strategies. Try asking, "Is there anything I can do when I'm there?" or "Is there anything I can take with me?" To elicit helpful thoughts, you can ask, "Is there anything I should remember?"

If you don't have other animals available, you can ask the wise owl for advice yourself. You may choose to ask about a worry as though it is yours, or you could ask for advice for another child who comes to see you. Alternatively, you could role play some animals and pretend you are visiting the owl for advice.

If the child is reluctant to have a turn at being the owl, you can be the owl first and then see if they are happy to have a go.

## What families can do

Reflect with parents on what a wise owl their child is. Encourage the child to take the owl home and suggest that parents ask their child about what a wise owl might say when they are having a difficult time managing their worries at home.

## Developmental considerations

Younger children and those with developmental difficulties are likely to come up with more simplistic strategies, whereas older children will tend to have more sophisticated strategies and a larger number of cognitive strategies. Ensuring that you are modeling developmentally appropriate strategies is important.

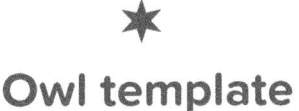

## Owl template

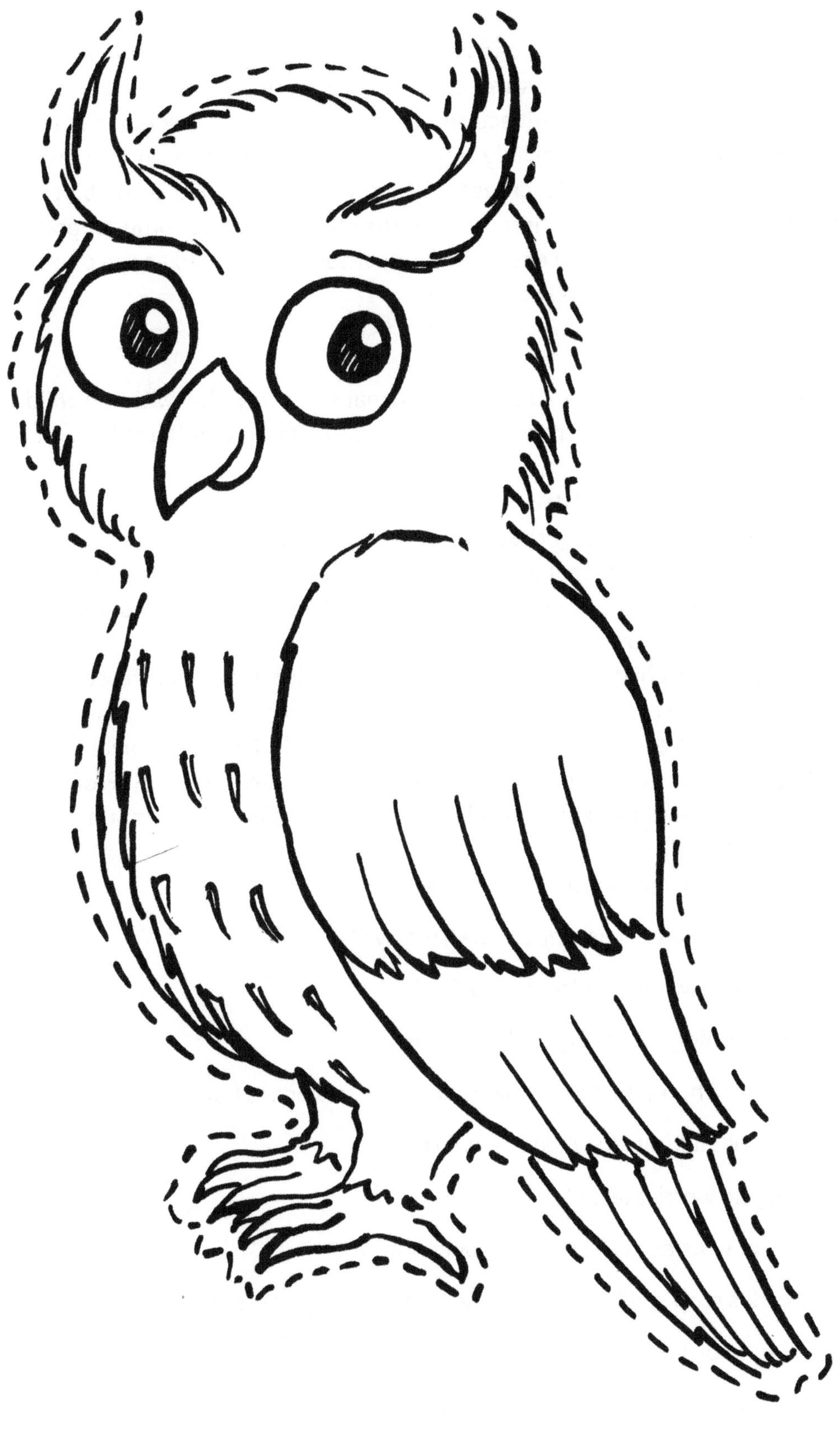

# Expert news report

This activity uses a narrative approach and helps children reflect on what they have learnt about worries and to generate or revise strategies that are useful for looking after themselves when they are worried. It helps children to reflect on how they experience anxiety in their body, the thoughts they tend to have, how they typically respond and what helps them to manage. It puts the child in the position of "expert" and increases their confidence in their own abilities. It is often best to use this activity some way into therapy when the child has made some progress and can reflect on this. It is also a lovely activity to end therapy, positioning the child as the one who has the answers rather than the one who needs the support.

## What you'll need

You will need a toy microphone. You may like to make this together with the child, using a cardboard tube and a ball of tin foil. Alternatively, you can use a plastic or inflatable microphone.

## Introducing this activity

Explain to the child and family that you have noticed that they have learnt some good ways of managing their worries. Say that you often see children who have similar difficulties and would love others to have all of their advice and wisdom about what they can do. Ask if you could interview them, like on the news, as a way of hearing all of their advice.

Suggest that the child might like to be someone else, maybe Professor Calm or Doctor Worry, or that they may like to be themselves. Put on a silly voice and, using the microphone, introduce the child. For example, you could say, "Good evening, all. This is Reporter Explorer reporting from Channel Y News. Many children suffer from worries. I'm here today with Professor Calm, who knows lots about worries and has some good ideas for how children can manage these. Thank you for joining us, Professor."

You can then ask lots of useful questions such as:

"Professor, can you tell us why children worry?"

"What happens when children worry?"

"Is there anything that happens in their bodies?"

"What sort of thoughts do they have when these worries happen?"

"What might children do when they worry?"

"How long do worries last?"

"How might worries get in the way for children?"

"Can worries stop children from doing things they want to do?"

"What would be your advice to children who worry?"

"What are some of the things children can do when they are worried?"

"Is there anything you'd like children who worry to always remember?"

"Is there anything parents can do to help?"

"What about teachers?"

## What families can do

Parents can easily be involved in the session and may like to watch the interview. You can also interview them as expert parents.

For parents who aren't able to attend the session, you may like to suggest that children take a microphone home and do the interview at home with them. You can also videotape the interview and share that with the parents as a way of including them in the activity.

## Developmental considerations

Younger children with good language skills can engage in this activity if you use very simple questions and keep it briefer. Questions that are narrower in focus are also best for this age group. For example, if you have been working with a child with a dog phobia, keep the questions related to fear of dogs specifically rather than worries more broadly.

More generally, it is important to consider a child's language abilities and modify your approach accordingly when using this activity. This will be particularly important when working with children with developmental difficulties.

# My treasures

Knowing what is important to a child is important in therapy. It helps children balance their thinking and often improves their mood. More specifically, it can help motivate children with anxiety to deal with their fears. For example, a child who treasures her friends but is anxious about going to school might find that getting to be with her friends makes it worth going to school.

## What you'll need

You will need some treasures for this activity. The treasures need to be something that the child can keep and take with them. Something that is shiny and jewel-like seems to work well. Small shiny pebbles (like those used in vases) work well, as do sequins. Having a variety of shapes, colors and sizes helps.

## Introducing this activity

Explain that you are curious about what is important to the child. What do they treasure? Suggest that you play a game so that you can learn about this. Have the treasures in a shallow bowl or tray and suggest that you take it in turns to choose one for each of the things in your life that you treasure.

Model this first if the child does not spontaneously engage in the task. For example, you might say that you treasure your family and choose a treasure to represent this. Then have the child take a turn. Some children will happily continue to choose gems and name what they treasure. Others will prefer to take it in turns.

Talk about each of the child's treasures as you label them. How does that treasure make them feel? Are there times when that treasure is really helpful? Is there anything that gets in the way of them enjoying that treasure? Would they like to have that treasure more often? How might this happen? What happens if they are worried and do something they treasure? Is the treasure worth experiencing some anxiety for? Often children find that it is worth sitting with some anxiety if it allows them to do what is important to them.

## What families can do

Parents often benefit from hearing about what is important to their child. Checking in about whether or not they knew this was a treasure to their child can be valuable as can eliciting their ideas about how their child can spend more time doing the things they treasure.

## Developmental considerations

Younger children may need you to give them more examples in order to support them to engage in this task. They are also likely to benefit from having some support from parents. Children with developmental difficulties may similarly need support to reflect on what they value. Starting with their special interests is often useful.

Older children are often able to think about their treasures with less support.

With all children, it is important to remember that a child's values are constantly changing and developing. For these reasons a child may like to complete this activity a number of times throughout therapy.

# What floats your boat?

Building a child's insight into what helps them feel relaxed and happy is valuable for all children, particularly those who are anxious. Regularly engaging in these activities helps to lower a child's overall stress levels and vulnerability to anxiety. Parents benefit from having a good sense of what relaxes their child as this can help them to regulate their child. Older children can begin to learn to do this for themselves too.

## What you'll need
You can use bamboo serving boats, which are available from kitchenware and discount stores. Alternatively, you could fold a simple boat out of paper for this activity (if you need instructions for folding it, you'll find some online). You will also need a sink or a tub of water to float the boat in.

## Introducing this activity
You can begin by saying to the child that you thought you would make some boats to play with today. Offer the child a bamboo boat and ask whether the child has ever heard the saying "Whatever floats your boat" and what they think it might mean.

If the child is not aware of the saying, explain that things that float your boat are those things that you enjoy, the things that help you feel happy and relaxed. Let the child know that these things are different for everyone and suggest you think together about what floats the child's boat.

As you talk about what floats the child's boat, record this by marking the bamboo or paper boat with permanent marker. For example, if the child loves to read, you might decide to name the boat *The Good Book* or *The Bookworm*. In addition to naming the boat, you can draw pictures or write words that symbolize what the child finds enjoyable and relaxing either inside or outside of the boat.

Talk with the child about what it feels like when they do something that floats their boat. What does their body feel like? What sort of thoughts do they have? What is a name for how they feel? Ask the same questions about what happens if they haven't been able to do anything that floats their boat.

Children often like to place their boats in water and try them out, so having a sink or a tub of water to float the boats in can be a fun idea. Keep in mind that if you are using a paper boat it will get soggy if you float it for too long, so you may need to talk with the child about this.

Older children may like to extend upon this activity by thinking about what sinks their boat. Having some stones that fit within the boat is a useful way of exploring this idea. You can write something that sinks a child's boat on each stone with permanent marker before placing it in the boat. For example, not having anyone to play with might be something that a child chooses to put on a stone. Some children will like to choose bigger stones for bigger challenges and smaller stones for smaller challenges.

## What families can do
If a parent is present during the session, they may like to make their own boat to float. If not, children are likely to enjoy showing their boat to parents later, or they may like to make a video of their boat floating to share with their parents. Taking the boat home is also a great idea to encourage children and families to think about these ideas further.

More generally, it is helpful for parents to understand that regularly engaging in activities that float their child's boat helps them to manage stress and anxiety. Parents can be encouraged to think about when the child can engage in these activities.

## Developmental considerations

Younger children would benefit from having parents in the session while you complete this activity so that you are able to talk to them about the importance of doing things that you enjoy and find relaxing. Drawing a picture (rather than using words) as a way of recording things that make them feel happy and relaxed is also useful for children in this age group.

# Shield ball

It is important for anxious children and their parents to have an understanding of their strengths, as anxiety can impact on their self-esteem. Strengths can also help a child to face their anxiety. This activity is an engaging way to highlight and reinforce a child's strengths and resources and explore how these can help when they face anxiety.

## What you'll need
You will need cardboard to make the shield (you can use the *Shield template* below printed onto cardboard), as well as markers. You will also need a small soft ball.

## Introducing this activity
Begin by talking with the child about some of the anxiety-provoking events you know they have faced lately and reflecting on how difficult that was. Ask the child about anything that helped them to manage these challenges and use this conversation to begin to draw out strengths and resources. Talk with the child about how we all have things we do well and how we have good things in our lives that make it easier when we are faced with a challenge. Explain that these form a kind of shield and suggest that together you make a shield so you can play with this idea.

Create a shield either by drawing one freehand or using the template below, talking about the child's strengths and resources as you do so. Some children may like to decorate the shield with their strengths and resources by drawing pictures of these or writing them down. For some children you might need to describe strengths that you have noticed, providing examples of these. Try to think broadly about strengths and resources, and include skills, strategies they have learnt, interests, activities they enjoy, people who are important to them, things they feel good about, and other things that are important to them.

Take your time exploring each of the strengths and resources that are identified and how the shield might be protective when the child is faced with anxiety. You might like to reflect on how many different strengths the child has, or how strengths are something that we develop and grow over time.

When the child is ready, suggest that you test it out. Have the child hold the shield and try to use it to protect themselves from the soft ball as you throw it at them. Talk about how the ball is a bit like an anxiety-provoking situation and notice that while the shield offers some protection it does not stop the ball from being thrown. Depending on your focus with the child, you may like to experiment with throwing the ball at them with and without the shield.

## What families can do
It is helpful for parents to be aware of their child's strengths and resources and to reinforce these at home. You may like to involve parents in the activity by asking them to help in identifying strengths that the child has, or they may be able to give examples of times they have seen their child using one of their strengths. They may be able to draw on the child's strengths in moments of anxiety. They can also reflect on what is important to the child and encourage the child to use these interests and

resources when they are anxious. Talk with the child and parent about where they might hang their shield ball at home as a reminder.

## Developmental considerations

Younger children will need their parents present to assist with identifying strengths and to continue to reinforce these ideas at home. Older children are better placed to consider their own strengths and may be able to complete the activity independently.

# Shield ball template

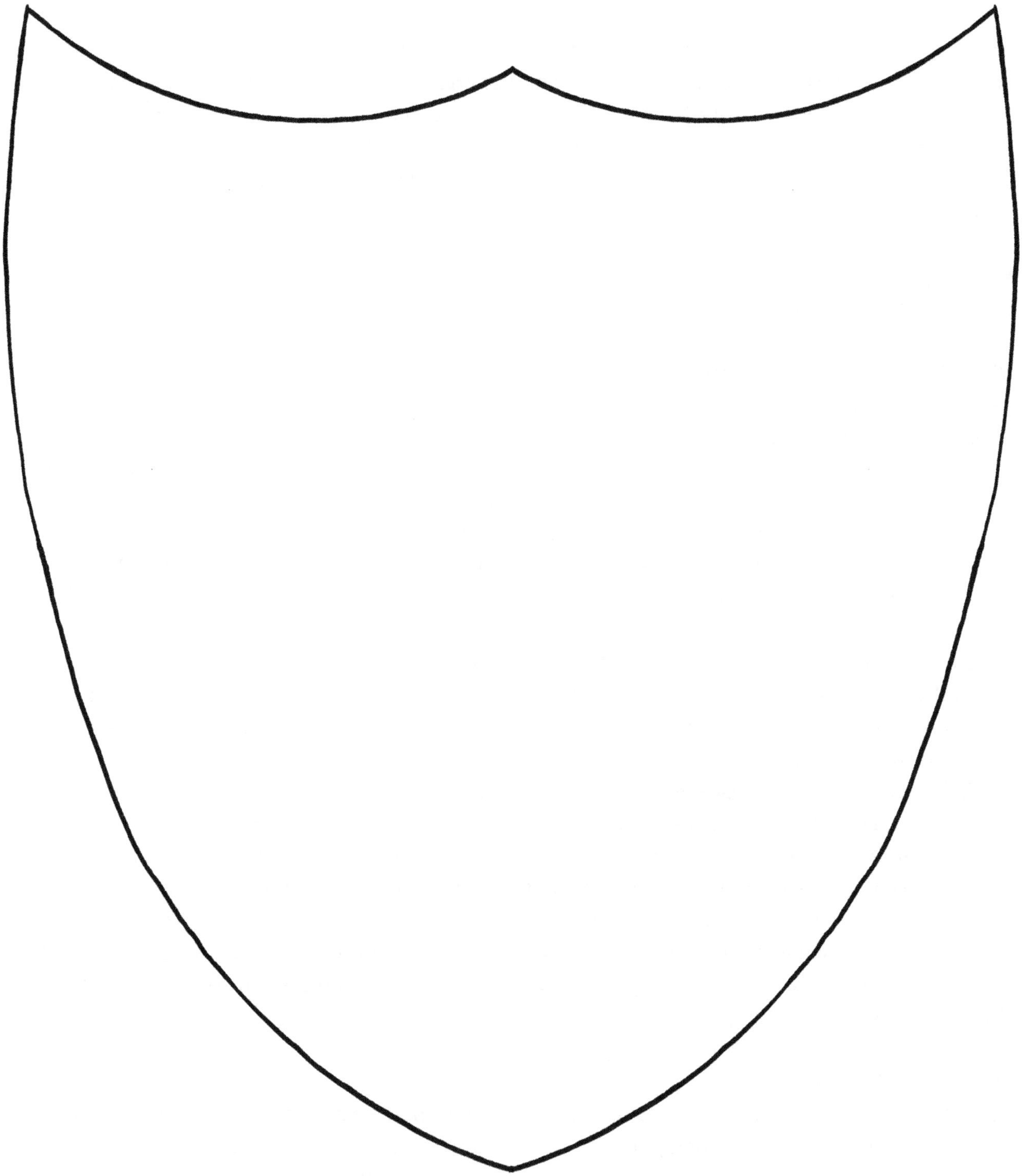

# Compliments box

Anxious children often have the experience of not doing the things that other children take for granted. They often underestimate their own abilities and their self-esteem can suffer. Their parents are often worried and frustrated and a child's strengths can go unnoticed. This is a simple activity that seeks to redress the balance. It can be used to help children reflect on their strengths and positive ways in which others view them as well as how their own positive thinking can impact on how they are feeling.

## What you'll need
You will need a box, paper and markers or a pen.

## Introducing this activity
Ask the child if they know what a compliment is. If they don't know, explain that it is when others tell us what they like about us or what we are good at or do well. You may like to describe a compliment someone gave you and what it felt like to hear them say that. Ask the child about a compliment someone has given them and what that felt like.

Talk about how hard it can be when things are difficult to remember those things that we are good at or do well. Suggest that it might be useful to write down some of the compliments the child has had so that they can keep these in a box for those difficult times. Choose a box with the child and begin writing the compliments down on pieces of paper and putting these inside the box.

Some children will find it hard to think about compliments they have received, so you may need to ask their parents to reflect on what others have said about their child over the years. If you don't have the parent in the room, encourage the child to think broadly—ask about what their friends say, what their teachers say and what their family members say.

Talk about how we can also compliment ourselves. We can notice when we have done something well and can acknowledge our strengths. Doing so often helps us to feel better. Check if there are any compliments the child has for themselves that they would like to put into the box. You may also have some compliments to put into the box for the child, based on what you know about them.

Encourage the child to reflect on what it felt like to write all of the compliments down. Notice what changes in their feelings, their body and with their thoughts. Wonder together about when the compliments would be most helpful and when the child might need them most. Talk about where the child might want to keep them.

## What families can do
Parents can join in this activity, making their own compliments box and adding to the child's compliments box. When involving parents, it's important to be mindful that some parents can find it difficult to accept compliments and can instead be openly dismissive of them. Supporting parents to model acceptance of compliments is helpful.

It is important for parents to understand how helpful it is to for them to notice and acknowledge their child's strengths in an ongoing way. If parents are not present for this activity, you can provide them with an explanation and ask that they add their own compliments, and compliments they have heard from others about their child, into the box later. The child can bring the box home to show their family, and further compliments can be added by family members.

## Developmental considerations
Both younger and older children can engage in this activity. Younger children will need a parent present to help them think of compliments they have received, as may children with developmental difficulties.

# Kicking toward my goal

This activity helps children understand the concept of moving toward their goals and what takes them closer as well as what might take them further away. It is a useful way of helping anxious children to think about their goal and how they can move toward this despite feeling anxious.

## What you'll need
You will need a soft ball for this activity.

## Introducing this activity
Ask the family if they have watched soccer and encourage them to explain how the game works to you. Elicit some discussion about the direction in which players kick the ball, clarifying that they kick toward their goal.

Reflect on a goal the child might have—something they might want. For example, this might be about wanting to learn how to swim despite being worried about the water; it might be something more general, like being able to be worried and still do the things they want to do; or it might be something more specific, like being able to sleep the night at a friend's place.

Set up a goal in the room and take out a soft ball. A simple way to create a goal is to use a table or the legs of a chair. Encourage the child to say one thing that helps and then have a go at kicking toward the goal.

Children will often miss the goal and this creates a good opportunity for discussion. It is worth reminding children that soccer is a very low-scoring game. You may like to look at some recent game scores online as a way of communicating this. Talk about how the important thing is that we are trying to kick toward our goals and how the child is more likely to get a goal if they are kicking the ball down that end of the field.

You can continue to play the game, each time asking the child to identify something that helps them move toward the goal they identified as they kick. This may provide an opportunity to reflect on how many different helpful moves the child has, or how sometimes trying the same move more than once can be helpful.

## What families can do
It is helpful for parents to have an understanding of the child's goals and actions that help them move toward those goals. Parents might have additional ideas of helpful moves that the child could consider, or they may be able to identify their own moves as teammates kicking toward the same goal. They can identify these moves by joining in the game and taking turns to kick, or through conversation later.

## Developmental considerations
Both younger and older children can engage in this activity. Younger children and those with developmental difficulties often choose a simple behavioral goal and are limited in the actions they can think of to move toward the goal, requiring parental assistance with this. Older children tend to choose goals that are more general and which may display some of their values. They can also generate more ideas for actions they can take and can have more independence in these actions.

# Putting it all together

Often there are many different aspects that go into managing a child's anxiety. Successful intervention often relies on both parents responding differently to the child, and children learning some strategies of their own. These pieces need to fit together, much in the way a jigsaw does, so this activity involves identifying all of the helpful pieces in their individual puzzle. Having a visual reminder of your strategies is often helpful, particularly toward the end of therapy when you are close to finishing up.

## What you'll need

You can buy pre-cut blank jigsaw puzzles from craft and discount stores. Alternatively, you can cut your own from cardboard. You might like to use the *Jigsaw puzzle template* below.

## Introducing this activity

Reflect on some of the changes you have noticed with the child. Say that you've noticed some of the things they have done and some of the things their parents have done, and that all of this seems to have come together and helped.

Suggest that it's been a bit like a jigsaw. Look at a blank jigsaw as you talk, noticing how each of the pieces is needed in order for the jigsaw to be complete. Working with the child, list something that has been helpful on each of the pieces. For example, this might include "Mom understanding what worries me" and "Having a go when I am worried."

When you have listed as many pieces as you can think of, turn the puzzle over and have the child draw a picture on the other side. This might be a picture of the child feeling relaxed or doing something they are able to do now that they are less worried.

Once the puzzle is complete, break it into pieces (or cut it up if you are using a cardboard one). Help the child to reassemble it, talking about each of the strategies as you put it together.

## What families can do

This is a great activity to complete with parents, acknowledging the helpful changes that they have made as well as their child and hearing their thoughts about what has been helpful. Alternatively, the child can show their parents the puzzle later and talk about the strategies they found helpful. You can give the child the puzzle to take home in an envelope and suggest that they look at some of the pieces with their parents when faced with future worries.

## Developmental considerations

For younger children and those with developmental difficulties the concept of all of the different strategies fitting together may be complex; however, you can focus on listing what has helped on the pieces. Completing this activity with the child's parents in the room should be helpful as it will allow the parents to have a good sense of what has helped and to feel prepared for future challenges. The puzzle itself also acts as a visual cue and is a good reminder of strategies for younger children.

# Jigsaw puzzle template

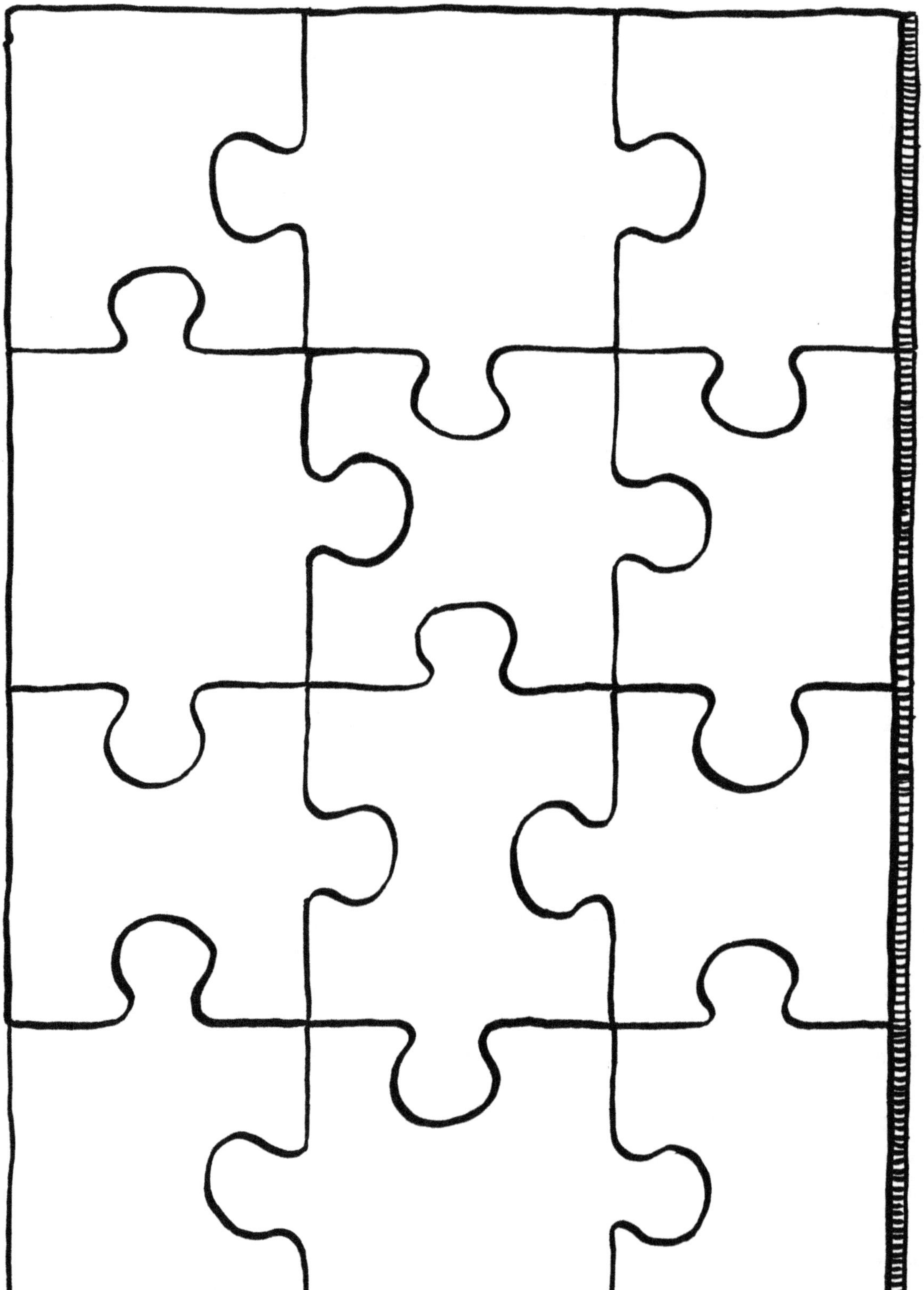

# Moves for life

Children who are anxious often struggle with problem-solving. Learning to respond thoughtfully when faced with anxiety-provoking situations, rather than simply reacting, is often a focus in therapy. This activity uses a popular children's game to help children discover the value of pausing and considering before acting and encourages them to think about how this might apply to their day-to-day life.

## What you'll need
This activity works well with a game of four-in-a-row such as Connect Four by Milton Bradley. If you don't have Connect Four or similar, you can use the paper and pencil game noughts and crosses or tic-tac-toe. These games are quick, allowing multiple trials, and they require players to consider not only their own tokens/moves but also their opponents'.

## Introducing this activity
Suggest to the child that you play Connect Four for a while. As you play, notice anything that the child does prior to taking a turn. For example, you might notice the child:

- pausing before placing their token

- taking some time to think before placing their token

- looking at the board to notice where your tokens are

- thinking about what you might be doing with your tokens

- thinking about where to place their token

- feeling anxious about where to place the token

- feeling disappointed or frustrated if you block their token

- feeling excited when they place a winning token.

It is also worth noticing and reflecting when you have the above experiences.

Once you have played one game, take some time to pause and ask the child what was helpful and make a list together. For example, this might be a "Before you move" list or a "Top tips for making good moves" list, depending on what the child wants to call it. It is essential to include on the list the need to pause and think before placing a token. Try, however, to keep the list limited to no more than three points as the idea is not to make problem-solving time-consuming or to add to the child's anxiety about making decisions; rather the idea is to reassure the child and create some helpful strategies for approaching challenges. Depending on the child and their specific presentation, you may also want to include aspects like noticing and naming feelings or thinking about what the other person is doing. Suggest that you keep the list handy while you play again.

As you play a second game, wonder about whether the list might be helpful in any other situations. Are there times when the child has used these strategies and found them to be helpful? For example, have there been situations in which they have been anxious and have found it useful to pause and think about what to do, or times when wondering about what another person might be thinking has helped? Are there times in the child's life where this could be useful? Reflect on some of the situations they feel worried in and check the list for any strategies that might help. If the child struggles to make this connection, you may want to draw on any recent situations you know they have faced and help them to think about how these strategies relate.

## What families can do

Where parents are present for the session, it can be useful to have them engage in a game or two and see if they can utilize the list of ideas for how to make good moves when playing. They can also help to reflect on times when the child has made good moves in their day-to-day life or when those ideas might be helpful for some of the situations their child is faced with.

It is helpful for all parents to be provided with an explanation of the list, so that they can gently encourage these strategies when relevant at home. The child can take the list home as a reminder of how they might be able to make good moves in life.

## Developmental considerations

This activity is suitable for typically developing children from around 7 years old. Older children will be able to identify more complex ideas around what helps when making a move and can generally generate more ideas. Younger children can benefit from this activity if you stick with a smaller number of ideas or even just one idea. Pausing and thinking is often the best idea to focus on.

# CHAPTER 7

# NOTICING, UNDERSTANDING AND MANAGING ANXIOUS THOUGHTS

### MUHAMMAD

Muhammad was a 6-year-old boy with separation and generalized anxiety. He was not yet able to identify thoughts when asked directly about these. The therapist was, however, able to model thoughts in the therapy session, saying, "I'm having the thought that…" The therapist chose to notice thoughts that were not emotionally laden or uncomfortable initially, with the purpose of tuning Muhammad into his thoughts in the first instance. He was able to pick up on this in the session and spontaneously began using "I'm thinking…," which supported him to engage further in work around thoughts.

In Chapter 1 we outlined the cognitive processes that are commonly seen in children with anxiety, noting that anxious children tend to focus on threat and overestimate the likelihood of something bad happening while underestimating their ability to cope. For example, Fliek *et al.* (2019) found that children who were anxious were more likely to have cognitive biases, such as perceiving ambiguous situations as threatening. In turn, however, these cognitive biases predicted higher levels of anxiety. Indeed, it is central to the cognitive behavioral model that how we think impacts how we feel and behave; and, in turn, how we feel and behave affects how we think.

Understanding the cognitive processes that are involved in a child's anxiety influences the way we work with them and their families. Often in our work with children we are helping them to see situations in a more balanced way, or we are helping parents to foster their child's belief in their own ability to cope.

Cognitive processes can change, and we know that doing things differently alters the way we think. Indeed, one key aspect of therapy is that behavior has the ability to change cognitions. In therapy we give children the opportunity to have different experiences with the knowledge that this is likely to change the way they think. Parents too have the chance to see their child in a different light or to engage with their child in a different way. Using play in therapy is a great way of creating experiences that allow us to think differently. Play provides children with the opportunity to explore another point of view and allows the child to have new experiences. For example, a child who is fearful of making mistakes can be encouraged to make mistakes in a playful way (i.e., in a game or drawing) to experience making mistakes and coping with them. This may challenge any beliefs they have about how bad it would be to make the mistake, and they may learn that their anxious feelings about this are manageable and pass quickly. *Scavenger hunt* (page 191) is an example of a therapeutic activity that provides a child who has separation anxiety with a playful experience of moving away from their parent, often eliciting feelings of enjoyment and happiness rather than anxiety. For children who do experience anxiety while engaged in this activity, it provides an opportunity to reflect on those times when it is worth doing the thing you are anxious about, such as separating from your parent in order to collect the item on your list and hopefully win the game.

One of the things we focus on in therapy is how parents interact with children and how this influences both the child's thoughts and their own. Often parents know the right words to say to children; however, their behaviors might not match. We often see parents reassuring their children that it will be ok but they look anxious and spend so much time providing reassurance that often the child gets the opposite message. It's important to talk with parents about the messages they want to convey to their children around their ability to have a go and manage any difficulties or anxious feelings that may come up. Reflecting on how they can do this both verbally and non-verbally is helpful.

When we are focussing more explicitly on thoughts in therapy with children, we find that just noticing thoughts is a good first step. Younger children are often not aware of their thoughts. They use self-talk, which is private speech spoken out loud, to guide their behaviour, and this becomes internalized between about 5 and 7 years of age. For both younger and older children, however, it is useful to introduce thoughts informally. We would tend to do this by noticing our own thoughts in sessions. For example, if we were trying to make something and the glue wasn't working, we might say, "I'm having the thought that we might need to use some sticky tape." This thought doesn't relate to the presenting difficulty and the reason the child is coming to therapy. Modeling thoughts that are not emotionally laden is a non-threatening way of introducing the concept of thoughts. Articulating our thoughts alerts the child to the presence of thoughts, which is a good way of preparing the child to work on thoughts in future.

The way in which we introduce thoughts is also important. In the example above, the function of the statement "I'm having the thought that…" is a way of distancing myself from the thought and fits within an ACT framework. ACT principles encourage us to think about thoughts as coming and going and this encourages us to become less fused with our thoughts. So, "I'm having the thought that…" is significantly different from "I'm thinking…" If you are working from an ACT framework, it is useful to use this language from the beginning of therapy. Other examples of language you could use about thoughts that fits within an ACT framework include "My mind is telling me that …" or "One of the thoughts in my head is that…" The activities *Catching thoughts* (page 165) and *Sometimes*

*I have the thought that…* (page 164) are helpful in supporting children to notice some of their thoughts and become less stuck to or fused with those thoughts.

One of the key features of thoughts is that they are transient—they come and go, much in the way that feelings do. This is an important tenet of ACT and is something that is often very helpful for children and families. Knowing that a really uncomfortable feeling and thought will pass often makes it more bearable for both the child and the parents. This is, however, quite an abstract concept, and explaining it to families often requires play to make it meaningful. In Zandt and Barrett (2017, p.130) we outline an activity called *Feelings bubbles*, in which we blow bubbles while speaking with the child about how feelings and thoughts are like bubbles. Some are big and some are small, some float farther away from us, and others stay close. Some last longer and others are gone sooner; however, they all pass at some point. It's important to acknowledge that some thoughts do stick around for a long time and to carefully validate children's experience of these.

Helping children to understand that we have a range of thoughts, that our thoughts can change, and that our thoughts can impact on how we feel and behave, can be important in therapy. This often includes exploring how some thoughts are helpful, in that they help us to feel better or to do the things that are important to us, whereas other thoughts might be unhelpful, adding to our worried feelings or stopping us from doing what we want or need to do. *Pet worry* (page 102) is one of our activities that can help children to understand these ideas. Developing a child's awareness of thoughts, and their understanding of how thoughts may or may not be helpful or comfortable, and that they will pass, are important first steps in cognitive work and may be enough for many children.

Encouraging helpful thoughts or positive self-talk is another cognitive strategy that can be useful for both younger and older children. This does not necessarily involve the child articulating or evaluating, or even being aware of their unhelpful thoughts. Children can learn to use helpful thoughts that are not directly related to their unhelpful thoughts. For example, a child who can use the helpful thought of "Everyone makes mistakes sometimes" is likely to be better able to manage work they perceive to be difficult. This is true regardless of their awareness of some of their unhelpful thoughts, which might include "My work needs to be perfect" and "Making mistakes is not ok." Keeping this in mind is particularly important with younger children who find it difficult to articulate their thoughts and have yet to develop the logical thinking capacity to engage in thought challenging. From a developmental perspective, younger children in the 4–6-year-old age group are still using private speech spoken out loud, so encouraging them to say the helpful thought out loud fits well. Some of the activities in this book are aimed at encouraging helpful self-talk and are well suited to this age group. These include *My cheer squad* (page 171), *Mom in my pocket* (page 173), *Positive paths* (page 174) and *Magic words* (page 175).

ACT and CBT differ in terms of how they suggest unhelpful or uncomfortable thoughts are managed. ACT emphasizes cognitive defusion; that is, ways in which the child can become less fused with the thought. The activity *Weaving thoughts* (page 169) helps children to carry their uncomfortable thoughts more loosely to reduce the impact of these thoughts. Other ways ACT therapists support children to do this are by singing their thought to a familiar tune or saying it in a funny voice (e.g., Hayes, Strosahl and Wilson 1999, cited in Harris 2019). We like to do this with older children using apps that change speech into a song or rap (e.g., AutoRap) or apps that change your voice in fun, silly ways (e.g., Talking Tom). We are careful to normalize the fact that we all have unhelpful thoughts, and that these are just thoughts that we can let come and go, or we can remember them in the funny voice or song. Some older children like to come up with a name for their unhelpful thoughts, such as "Old Mr. Worry," and either find a voice on the app to match Old Mr. Worry or create the Old Mr. Worry Rap. They can then respond to their thoughts with "Oh, that's just Old Mr. Worry again" or "Yes, thank you, Old Mr. Worry."

Within a traditional CBT approach, cognitive restructuring involves identifying thoughts that are associated with the anxiety and evaluating how useful and accurate these thoughts are (Hudson *et al.* 2019). This type of cognitive restructuring work is generally less of a feature in child therapy because children often can't articulate and evaluate their thoughts in the way that adults can. Younger children are still developing their cognitive abilities, and the best way to challenge their thoughts is through play with lots of guidance and input from the therapist. For example, for a child who is anxious about the water, the therapist might use puppet play, using a puppet to articulate some thoughts about the water that the child can use another puppet to challenge. The therapist's puppet might say something like "I'm worried I might get water in my eyes and it might sting" or "What if the water is over my head?" The child's puppet might share their experience that gently challenges the thoughts of the therapist's puppet. *Wise owl* (page 142) is a more structured version of this sort of play and is useful for both younger and older children.

Older children are much more able to logically challenge some of their thoughts though they still need support from the therapist in order to be able to do so. The therapist will often need to provide structure for children, helping them clearly articulate some of their unhelpful thoughts, look for the evidence and re-evaluate. Asking children questions such as "What would you say to a friend who was feeling worried and thinking this?" can be helpful in generating a different perspective. An activity in this book that supports children to challenge their thoughts is *On the plus side* (page 178).

Some older children may also be interested in learning about common unhelpful thinking patterns or cognitive errors that can contribute to anxious feelings. We've outlined some of these patterns (which we've adapted from Stallard 2002 and Bunge *et al.* 2017) and presented a fun way to explore them in the activity *Thought error lotto* (page 180). Our aim in teaching these is to build the child's awareness of their patterns of worried thoughts and their understanding that their thoughts may or may not be accurate or helpful. We might simply encourage the child to notice when one of these worried thoughts pops into their mind, or to name the thought error (e.g., "There I go mind-reading" or "That's some black and white thinking right there"). This can help the child to distance themselves from the thought and to evaluate the thought. The activity *Tunnel vision worry* (page 110) can also be used to explore thinking errors relevant to a child and to challenge these thoughts.

Some therapists view CBT and ACT as very different and find it difficult to incorporate the two. There are certainly key differences in these therapeutic approaches; however, there are also many similarities, with ACT being a specific type of CBT. In practice we find that we can use components of the two quite comfortably, being guided by what works for the child and family. For example, we would often take an ACT approach, helping the child to notice thoughts and to realize that thoughts can be comfortable or uncomfortable and that they come and go. We then often do some work that aims to help a child unhook themselves from the thoughts, and sometimes this is where our therapy ends. At other times, however, children seem interested and capable of challenging their thoughts more directly and so we engage in some more direct challenging of thoughts.

# Sometimes I have the thought that...

This is a helpful activity for unsticking children from their thoughts and making the thoughts less powerful. The use of the word "sometimes" is helpful in that it implies flexibility, whereas words like "always" can indicate rigid thinking patterns. Similarly, the use of the phrase "Sometimes I have the thought that..." distances the child from the thought more than "I'm thinking..."

## What you'll need
You will need a game of four-in-a-row such as Connect Four by Milton Bradley.

## Introducing this activity
Explain to the child that you would like to play a game of Connect Four; however, suggest that you play a different version. Say that for every token each of you place, you will use the sentence stem "I sometimes have the thought that..."

You can go first, picking up a piece and completing the sentence stem. Keeping the first examples simple and less emotionally heavy can be useful until the child gets the idea. For example, you say, "Sometimes I have the thought that Connect Four is a really cool game."

Once the child understands how this works, you can move into more emotional examples. Try to choose examples that relate to the child. These might include:

- "I sometimes have the thought that I might get it wrong."

- "I sometimes have the thought that people think I'm silly/crazy/uncool."

- "I sometimes have the thought that I'm not good enough."

If the child struggles to come up with a thought, you might suggest one that they might experience (given your knowledge of them) and check if they ever experience that thought.

## What families can do
Parents may like to join in this game during the session, or they may be able to model using this sentence stem at home with their child. They can also be encouraged to respond to their child when they are upset by saying, "I'm wondering if you are having some thoughts about what happened?" or "I'm wondering if you are having the thought that..."

## Developmental considerations
Younger children are likely to find this activity challenging as they have a limited awareness of their own thoughts. It can be useful for increasing flexibility in a younger child though if you play this game using the sentence stem "I sometimes..." as it promotes the idea that the child can behave in different ways. Children with developmental difficulties may need more examples and opportunities for practice.

# Catching thoughts

This is a simple activity that increases a child's awareness of their thoughts and allows you to introduce the idea that thoughts are just thoughts.

## What you'll need
You will need some cotton balls and some small plastic scoops. The ones that come in boxes of washing powder are an ideal size—simply wash and dry before use—or you could use serving scoops made for candy jars.

## Introducing this activity
Talk with the child about thoughts, describing some examples of a thought. Try to include some thoughts that are comfortable (e.g., "I am good at this"), neutral (e.g., "I might need to try a different way") and some that are uncomfortable (e.g., "I am hopeless at this") when providing examples. Explain that we all have thoughts all of the time, though they can be hard to catch.

Suggest that you have a go at catching cotton balls in the scoops and talk about how these are difficult to catch too. Once the child has had a go at this, you can suggest that you say a thought each time you throw a cotton ball. Using a sentence structure like "Sometimes I have the thought that…" or "One of my thoughts is…" often helps as it implies some distance from the thought and emphasizes that thoughts are just thoughts. The child may like to throw the cotton ball thoughts for you to catch. Alternatively, you may like to throw cotton ball thoughts for the child to catch. Ideally, it is great to be able to take turns with this so that you have a chance to model and the child has a chance to reflect on some thoughts of their own.

Catching the cotton balls in a plastic scoop is difficult for most children and therapists and it provides a useful space to reflect on just how difficult it is to catch thoughts. Indeed, you may be able to notice the child feeling frustrated and reflect on some of their thoughts that are associated with this. It's also useful to notice how many thoughts there are and that they keep coming. Try experimenting and see if you are more likely to catch the thoughts if they are thrown slowly or if you throw them quickly. Is it easier or harder if there are lots of thoughts being thrown at you all at once?

Ask the child about whether there are any situations in which it is really hard to catch their thoughts. How could they slow down in these contexts and try to notice their thoughts, catching them like they have in the activity? Children may like to take away a scoop and some cotton balls so that they can continue playing with this at home and can show their parents.

## What families can do
Parents can join in the activity, or you can discuss the activity with them later, talking to them about how thoughts can impact on anxiety and how simply noticing thoughts can be helpful. Encouraging parents to share their own thoughts at home using a sentence similar to the above can be useful, as can having them guess at what their child might be thinking. For example, a parent might be able to say, "I'm wondering if you might be having the thought that you won't be able to do it. I sometimes have that thought too."

## Developmental considerations

This activity is useful for children 7 years of age and over, who should be able to notice their thoughts. For children who have developmental difficulties, you will need to have a good understanding of the child's language abilities and their awareness of their own thoughts before considering this activity. Introducing the idea of thoughts slowly and providing lots of opportunities for talking about comfortable and neutral thoughts initially can help, as can using some visuals to explain what thoughts are. Having a list of thoughts the child may have acts as a good starting point.

For younger children, activities that focus on private speech will be more developmentally appropriate than this activity.

# Pom pom thoughts

Often, children who are worried struggle with anxious thoughts. Some children will get caught up in the need to challenge these thoughts and can find the process exhausting and endless. For many children, learning that thoughts come and go is useful. This activity focusses on helping children to feel less bothered by their worried thoughts and to continue engaging in activities while they have worried thoughts.

## What you'll need

For this activity you will need a large number of pom poms. These are available from craft stores and come in a range of sizes. It is useful to have a selection of bigger and smaller ones. You will also need some paper and some pencils or markers.

## Introducing this activity

Begin by empathizing with the child about their many worried thoughts and their struggles to know how best to respond to these. Suggest that together you play a game to explore this further. Take out the pom poms and explain that you are going to pretend these are thoughts. You can list a few of the worried thoughts that the child has while looking at the pom poms. You may like to use a larger pom pom as an example of a big worried thought the child has and a smaller one as an example of a little worried thought the child has.

Explain that you'd like the child to do a drawing while at the same time hitting away all the pom poms, which you will be throwing at the child much in the way that worried thoughts come at them. The child can draw whatever they like; however, they have to hit away all of the pom poms. Agree that you will do this for a set amount of time: two minutes often works well. Once the time starts, throw the pom poms repeatedly at the child while they are drawing. You can label them as thoughts as you throw them, saying something like "Here comes a really big worried thought," or you can state worried thoughts that are similar to what the child experiences. For example, you can throw one pom pom saying, "What if no one talks to me" and another saying, "What if I make a mistake?" Whichever strategy you choose, it is important that you maintain a good pace of throwing and remind the child to continue hitting the pom poms away. At the end of the set time, stop throwing and reflect on what this felt like for the child. Wonder about whether their feelings changed as the thoughts continued to come at them. Look at their drawing and reflect on their experience of trying to draw while continually hitting the thoughts away.

After some reflection, suggest that you try a different approach. Suggest that this time the child allows the pom poms to hit them (reminding them that this won't hurt) and continues with their drawing. Repeat the process as above, throwing the pom poms repeatedly at the child and using them to represent the child's thoughts. Reflect again when the time is up about what that experience was like for the child. It is often helpful to talk about how their feelings changed over the time you were throwing the pom pom thoughts as many children will feel annoyed initially but this feeling will lessen as you keep throwing.

Help the child to compare their experience of needing to hit the thoughts away as opposed to letting them come and go. Look at the two drawings and ask what they notice about the pictures. Which picture is more complete? Which looks better?

Talk with the child about those times in their life when they notice the worried thoughts. What would happen if they let the thoughts come and go rather than feeling the need to challenge or hit these away? What might this be like for them? How hard might this be to begin with and would this be likely to change over time?

If the child is worried about you throwing pom poms at them during this activity, you may like to see if they can throw the pom pom thoughts at you while you do the drawing.

## What families can do

Parents can also become anxious about their child's anxious thoughts and try to stop the thoughts or to challenge them through excessive reassurance. It is helpful for parents to explore the idea that thoughts are transient and that it can be helpful to just notice the anxious thoughts and let them come and go again, while continuing to engage in important activities.

If family members are present when you use this activity, you can engage them in throwing worried thoughts. Alternatively, they may like to have a turn with you and the child throwing the worried thoughts at them. Otherwise, it is helpful to show the parents the pictures and provide an explanation about the activity and the therapeutic ideas.

## Developmental considerations

Children need to be aware of their thoughts in order to engage in this activity and to have articulated some of their worried thoughts. It is not necessary for children to be able to identify all of their worried thoughts, but understanding the concept is essential. As such, this activity may not be appropriate for younger children, and those with developmental difficulties may require some extra support.

# Weaving thoughts

This activity explores the idea of being able to hold our thoughts more loosely and how this might impact on how we feel.

## What you'll need
You will need sheets of different colored paper and some markers.

## Introducing this activity
Start by talking with the child about some of the uncomfortable thoughts you have noticed they have and suggest you do some experimenting with these thoughts. Cut some strips of paper and write some uncomfortable thoughts on the paper. Give a strip to the child and encourage them to reflect on how they feel holding that thought. Wonder about how they might feel if they carried that thought with them all day.

Explain that we can't always get rid of our unhelpful thoughts though we might be able to hold them less tightly. Suggest that you do something different with the thoughts and fold another piece of paper in half, cutting lines into it so that when you open it up it has cut lines that go through the middle with the borders intact. Take one of the thoughts and begin weaving it through the paper. This should mean that you can only see part of the thought.

Have the child try to read the thought you have woven through the paper. Because only part of the thought will be visible, doing so will often be a funny experience. Have them hold the paper with the thought woven through and reflect on what it would be like to hold onto this all day. Would that feel different to when they were holding the thought in the other way and if so, why?

Weave some of the other thoughts through the paper, repeating the process. Talk about how when we see thoughts as just thoughts and as part of our lives they can be less upsetting.

## What families can do
It is useful for families to understand the concept that thoughts are just thoughts. They can talk with children about this at home, saying things like "I'm wondering if you are having that 'I can't do it' thought again."

Parents can suggest worried thoughts or may like to weave a worried thought of their own in this activity. They can have a go at trying to read the woven thoughts and reflect on what it might feel like to carry those with them.

## Developmental considerations
Identifying thoughts is difficult for younger children, so this activity is better suited to older ones. Children with developmental difficulties may find this helpful; however, you may need to make some adaptations. For example, having a list of thoughts that the child can choose from may be easier than asking them to generate their own.

# Messages I receive

This activity helps children reflect on the messages they receive from others as well as from society more generally. It uses the metaphor of a mobile phone and is aimed at children toward the upper end of primary school. It encourages children to evaluate these messages in a more critical manner and to develop their own beliefs or more helpful ways of thinking. This is particularly helpful for anxious children who may be believing messages that contribute to their anxiety.

## What you'll need

You will need markers and a piece of cardboard or a sheet of craft foam, which you will use to make a phone. You might like to copy the *Phone template* on page 95.

## Introducing this activity

Talk with the child about how many messages you get on your phone. Talk about how these are both helpful and unhelpful. Reflect on how you get messages from friends and family as well as alerts about a broad range of things, from sales coming up to things that have happened in the news. Check that the child has understood this. If they have their own phone, ask about the messages they get or the messages their parents get.

Talk about how children get all sorts of messages. For example, they might get a message from watching TV or from social media that it is important to always have the latest clothes or always look perfect or to always be having fun. They might get messages from their parents or friends about how they should look or act. Check with the child about what sort of messages they feel they receive.

While you are talking, make a mobile phone together. Cut a phone shape out of cardboard or craft foam or use the *Phone template* on page 95. List some of the messages on the screen, reflecting on which messages the child hears most often and wondering about whether they are helpful or unhelpful. Wonder with the child about whether any of the messages add to their anxiety. Ask about which messages they would like the phone to be on silent for. Ask which messages they would like to ignore and what would happen if they did. Wonder together about whether they would do things differently if they did ignore these messages.

Often messages from society more generally are easier to identify. Some children, however, may be able and willing to talk about the messages they get from their parents or friends.

## What families can do

You can involve parents in the session. This is particularly helpful if you think that the child is not able to identify some of the messages they might be receiving. Alternatively, talking with parents afterwards about the messages their child gets, and from whom, is helpful. You may also be able to talk about the messages the child is getting from their parents.

## Developmental considerations

The concepts covered in this activity mean that it is more appropriate for older children—those toward the end of primary school. Younger children and older children with developmental difficulties may find this too challenging.

# My cheer squad

This activity helps children and families to understand the relationship between thoughts and feelings, and how helpful thoughts can be used in managing their anxiety. It is also a useful activity for engaging the family more broadly around worries.

## What you'll need
You will need crepe paper ribbon/streamers, scissors and sticky tape.

## Introducing this activity
Ask the family about the sporting teams they support and wonder if they have seen cheer squads. Talk about the role of a cheer squad and wonder about how the players might feel having people cheering for them. Encourage the child to think about what it might feel like if they were to have a group of people cheering for them. Talk about the importance of the words they might be saying and also what it might feel like to know that you have people on your side. Explain that sometimes families can be like cheer squads and that sometimes we can also cheer for ourselves by saying helpful words out loud or in our minds.

Suggest that you make some pom poms together so that you can think about cheering. The easiest way to make a pom pom is to take the crepe paper ribbon and ask the child to hold out an arm, bending it upwards at the elbow. Begin by winding the ribbon from the child's elbow up to their hand, having them grasp the ribbon as you do so, creating loops with the ribbon. Continue winding until you have wound the ribbon repeatedly around and then carefully slide the ribbon loops off the child's arm. Wrap some sticky tape around one end to bind the pom pom together. Use scissors to slit the ribbon at the other end (see Figure 7.1).

When the pom pom is complete, choose a situation and ask the child and the family to cheer for someone who might be in this situation. What would they say? Encouraging the child to wave and cheer noisily is often fun. Once you have used a few examples, you can choose something that relates to a situation the child feels anxious about. If the child's family are not present, you could have the child imagine their family as cheerleaders and reflect on what they might say. Ask about how others could cheer for them as well as how they might be able to cheer for themselves. Talking about how to cheer for yourself, either out loud or silently in your head, will assist the child to use positive self-talk when they feel anxious.

This activity can also be used to explore the role of unhelpful thoughts by having people use reverse cheering, saying things like "You'll never be able to do it." You can also use this activity for scaling by asking how loud or how long the cheer squad would need to cheer for the child to feel like they could face what they are worried about.

## What families can do
This is a great activity to do in the room with families. You can talk about when they might use their cheers and where at home they might keep their pom poms. You can suggest the family make a poster depicting their favorite cheers to display at home.

If parents are not present in the session, you could video the child chanting their favorite cheers to send to the parent along with an explanation of the activity, including the importance of positive self-talk in managing anxiety. The child might be happy for the parent to notice when they need a cheer and to prompt the child with "I wonder what cheer you could chant to yourself right now?" or to support them in saying one.

## Developmental considerations

This activity is appropriate for both younger and older children. For younger children, it will be important to have simpler cheers and to encourage them to say these cheers out loud, rather than expecting them to be able to say the cheers silently in their heads.

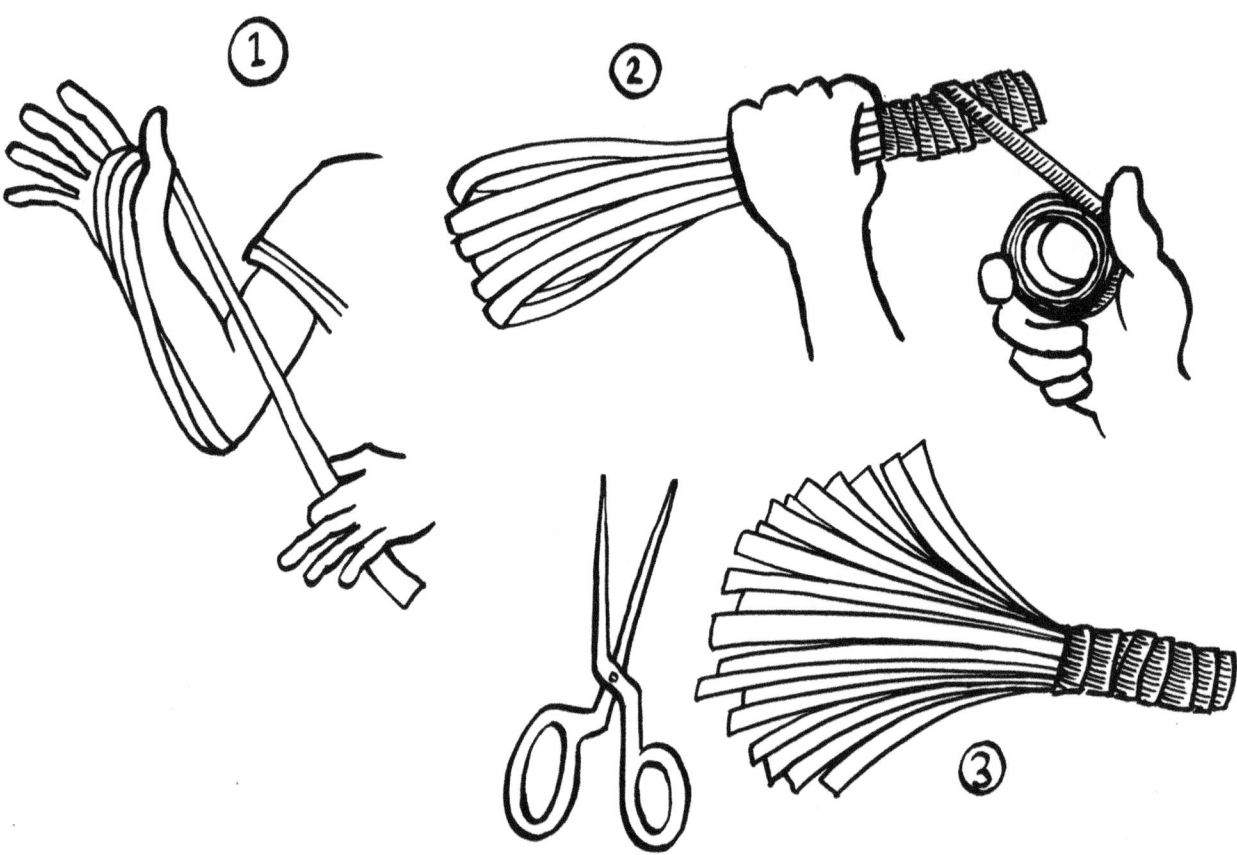

FIGURE 7.1 HOW TO MAKE A CHEERLEADING POM POM

# Mom in my pocket

This activity helps children develop positive self-talk and can reduce the amount of reassurance they seek. It also provides a nice way of helping children feel connected to their parents even in situations where they are not physically present, which can be useful if a child is experiencing separation anxiety.

## What you'll need
You will need a craft foam sheet or a piece of cardboard, scissors and markers.

## Introducing this activity
Talk with the child about how it sounds like Mom or Dad have lots of helpful things to say when they are feeling worried. Ask the child how it makes them feel to hear those things and wonder about what it would be like to have Mom or Dad in their pocket.

Suggest that you make a little Mom or Dad figure that could go in the child's pocket. Make a small figure out of cardboard or craft foam, having the child draw and then cut it out. Pop it into the child's pocket and talk about what it will be like to have Mom or Dad in their pocket. When might this be most helpful? What would Mom or Dad say in this situation?

You may like to write some of the helpful things Mom or Dad say on the back for the child so that they can more easily remember these.

## What families can do
Having a parent in the room is often helpful, particularly if a child is struggling to identify what Mom or Dad might say. Sometimes children might like their parent to write a special message for them each day as they head out to preschool or school, giving it to the pocket Mom or Dad to look after.

## Developmental considerations
Younger children find this activity enjoyable and the figure serves as a visual prompt that helps them to use positive self-talk out loud. Drawing a picture to go with the message from their parent is often helpful for younger children. Younger children may also benefit from having a preschool teacher read the words out loud to them, as hearing the words and speaking them out loud is most beneficial for this age group.

Older children may prefer a smaller version of this, such as notes scribbled on tiny pieces of paper, allowing them to keep it more private.

# Positive paths

This activity helps children explore the relationship between thoughts and feelings, and how helpful thoughts can assist us to feel less anxious and to do the things that are important to us.

## What you'll need
You will need paper or cardboard, and markers or a pen.

## Introducing this activity
Let the child know that you have been wondering about some of the thoughts they've mentioned and how these thoughts might help with their worries. Suggest that you make a pathway of positive thoughts and see what happens when the child walks along it.

Lay sheets of paper along the floor and have the child stand at one end. Ask about how they are feeling in that moment and have them show you what this feeling looks like. Together, come up with some helpful thoughts and write these down, one on each sheet. Suggest that the child walk the path, saying each of these thoughts aloud as they do so. When they reach the end, reflect on how they are feeling now and on how this looks in their body. Encouraging the child to experience their feelings by showing you what they look like should help them to connect the activity with their experiences.

You can add to the conversation by wondering about what they might do differently if they had to do something anxiety-provoking, like going to school or going upstairs on their own at home. What would it be like to need to do that before having walked the path? Would it be different if they had just walked the path?

## What families can do
Families can be included in this activity and may help to generate some helpful thoughts. They may have examples of times when positive thinking really helped them in their own journey.

If the child's parents are not present when you complete the activity, you can show them the path later and have them walk it with their child. Asking them to notice helpful thoughts at home should help, and the family may like to take the path home and display it there.

## Developmental considerations
This activity can be done with younger and older children. Using more general thoughts with young children is likely to help, such as "I can do it" or "I can have a go," as they are likely to find these thoughts easier to generalize. Younger children should also be encouraged to say these words aloud as they may still be using private self-talk rather than inner speech. With older children the complexity of the discussion you can have around this activity will obviously increase.

# Magic words

This is a great activity for helping children to better understand the role of helpful thinking and can be used to increase their repertoire of helpful thoughts. It can also be used in the context of values work, helping children to identify attributes such as courage that they would like to work toward.

## What you'll need
You will need a glue stick, a large sheet of cardboard and glitter. If you don't have cardboard, you could use poster paper.

## Introducing this activity
Talk with the child about how helpful words can be. Provide an example so that the child knows what you mean. For example, you might talk about a time when you felt scared and told yourself it would be ok. Ask the child whether there are any words that they aspire to when they are worried or any helpful thoughts that assist them. Talk about how powerful these words can be and how even though you can't see them they can make things happen. Explain that these words can be magical—they can change the way we feel. Talk to the child about how sometimes this might be a word (e.g., "breathe" or "courage") and other times it might be a thought (e.g., "I've done tricky things before"). Suggest that together you make a poster as a reminder of this.

Taking a glue stick, have the child write the word/helpful thought on a large sheet of cardboard. Talk about how we remember these words in our heads and others can't see them, just like they can't see the glue on the paper.

Explain that these words sometimes change what we do, which is something that can be seen. Shake some glitter over the glue as a way of making the word visible. Shake the excess into a container or bin, allowing the word to show.

Talk about the power of that word/thought and how magical it can be, and discuss when the child might be able to use that word/thought. Talk about where they might keep their poster to assist them to remember the word/thought.

## What families can do
If families are present in the session, they may like to make their own poster of helpful thoughts/words that they aspire to. Often children internalize what their parents say, so having parents in the room is a good way to think about positive words they use in their family. If families are not present when you complete the activity, it is helpful to speak with them about the value of words and show them the child's magic words poster.

## Developmental considerations
Older children are more likely to identify words that are meaningful to them as their more extensive vocabulary allows them to use more sophisticated language. Words like "courage" are more likely to hold meaning for them and may also be attached to memories that are helpful to reflect on.

Younger children are more likely to connect with simple phrases, such as those their parents might say to them. Choosing phrases that are simple and can be used in a range of situations is likely to assist generalization.

# Framing it

Children with anxiety often focus on their uncomfortable feelings and thoughts and those aspects of their life that are difficult or upsetting. This activity helps them to think about how they can choose their focus and understand the impact this has on how they feel.

## What you'll need

You will need paper and a pen or markers. You may like to print the *Frame templates* below onto cardboard to cut out. You may also like to use the brain from the *Time-traveling brain template* (page 141), enlarging it to A4 size, or you can draw this.

## Introducing this activity

Begin the activity by talking about the camera roll on your phone. Talk about how every time you look through it you see lots of great photos; however, there may be many more that are blurred or are even accidental photos of the ground. They are mostly all ok photos, but only a small number are worth framing.

Talk about how our minds are a bit like this. We have all sorts of thoughts, feelings and memories. Draw an outline of a brain or print an enlarged version of our brain template. List inside the brain some of the thoughts, feelings and memories that the child has. Talk about how some of those memories and thoughts are stronger and last longer, whereas others come and go more quickly.

Ask the child about which thoughts, feelings and memories they would most like to focus on, using the metaphor of choosing something to frame. Allow the child to choose a small frame cut out of cardboard and ask them to move it around on the brain to the thoughts, feelings or memories they would choose to frame.

You might also like to ask whether there are thoughts, feelings and memories that they frame sometimes that lead them to feel more worried. You can then discuss how choosing to frame other thoughts might help them to feel differently.

## What families can do

Parents can easily participate in this activity, thinking about which of their thoughts they would most like to frame. If parents don't participate, it is still helpful for them to understand the metaphor and the concept so they can refer to it in conversations at home. Children can take their drawing and frame home so that they are able to show and share it with other family members.

## Developmental considerations

Younger children may find this concept too abstract when linked to the brain and their thoughts. They may instead like to create a memory board or collage consisting of photos, certificates, letters, tickets and the like. Encourage them to choose memories that bring them joy—those they would most like to frame. Parents will be needed to assist with identifying and collecting the materials.

Older children can engage well in this activity and the concept of choosing which thoughts they would most like to frame. Some older children may like to create a camera roll of their own on their camera, tablet or other device, again including those things that help them to feel safe, calm and happy, and considering which ones they would most like to frame.

# Frames template

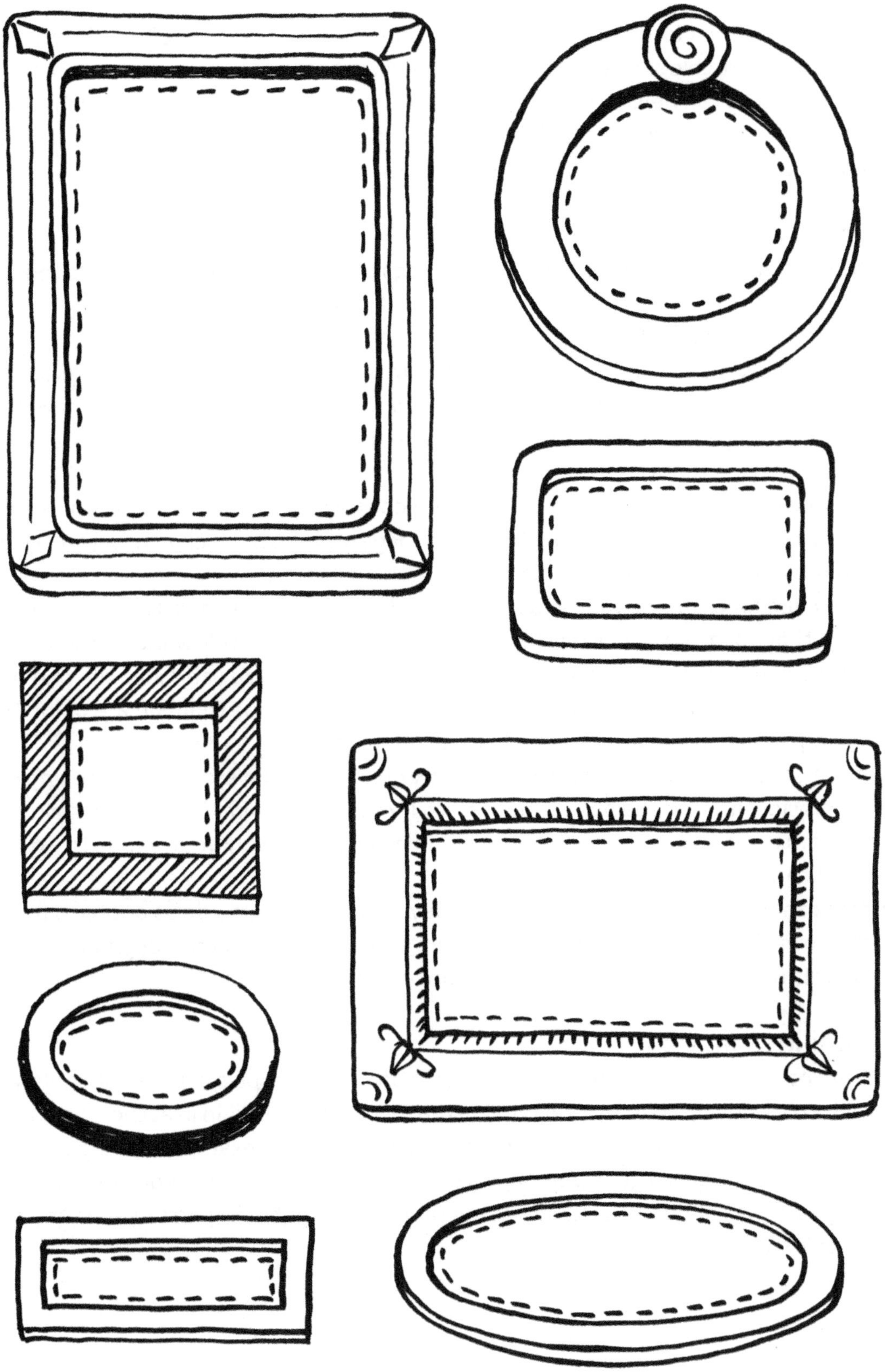

# On the plus side

This activity requires children to think about the positive aspects of a given situation (anxious children often have trouble seeing the positives). Helping them to do so can promote more balanced thinking. This activity can help children to manage situations they can't change, such as needing to do their work in class or needing to finish playing a video game. It can also be useful for engaging children in conversations about how our point of view relates to how we feel.

## What you'll need
You will need a large piece of cardboard and some pegs that can be easily attached to the cardboard.

## Introducing this activity
Explain to the child that you understand that there are some things that are really difficult for them to manage. Say that unfortunately some of those things are things that they just have to do. Give the child some examples of this. Suggest to the child that you play a game to think about the plus side in some of these situations.

Take a large piece of cardboard and draw a line down the middle of it. Draw a plus sign on one side and a minus sign on the other side. Take some pegs and show the child how you can peg them either onto the plus side or the downside (side with the minus sign).

Give the child an example while you show them how to use the pegs. For example, you might tell the child that you tried a new recipe on the weekend and it didn't work, while showing them the side of the card that has the minus sign marked on it. Then you can move the peg over to the plus side, explaining that on the plus side you found a better recipe that you are going to try next time. Thinking of one downside and one plus side is enough.

When the child has understood the concept, try giving them an example and seeing if they can think of a plus side, moving the peg as they do so. Try something simple like Mom saying she's run out of ice cream and so you can't have any after dinner, and then work your way up to examples that are pertinent to the child's anxiety.

Children can reflect on how they feel when they look on the plus side as opposed to when they look on the downside. Depending on where you are at with the child in therapy, you may like to link this to how this feels in their body or what they are thinking.

## What families can do
If parents are present in the session, they may like to provide examples of times when they have had to look on the plus side and have a go at moving the peg over. If they join in at the end of the session, then the child can demonstrate how this works and give them an example. Having the family take home the card and a peg is a good way of providing them with a reminder of this, and parents can be encouraged to ask about what the plus side might be after having first calmed their child and empathized with their feelings.

## Developmental considerations

Some younger children or those with developmental difficulties might find this activity challenging; however, it may still be useful to engage the family in this. Parents are often able to model what the plus side might be and, provided they do so having first acknowledged the child's feelings and are mindful of the downside, this can be helpful. For example, a parent who can say "I know it's annoying to have to stop when you are enjoying your game, but on the plus side we can go to the park now" is modeling some useful coping strategies for a child.

# Thought error lotto

Helping children to understand some of the thinking errors we can make when we are anxious is often helpful. This activity provides a hands-on way of introducing this idea.

## What you'll need

You will need cardboard to print four copies of the *Thought error lotto template* provided below onto some light card. Some children may like to decorate or color the game pieces with pencils or markers.

## Introducing this activity

Begin by talking with the child about some of the worried thoughts they have and explain that there is often a pattern with worried thoughts. Suggest that you make a game which will allow you to think about this. Use two of the template copies as a lotto board for each of you, giving one to the child and keeping one for yourself. With the remaining two copies, cut out the individual cards to use for the game.

As you cut out the cards to prepare the game, talk about the thought errors. For each thought error, provide an example and a brief description (as listed on the card). For example, introduce the idea of mind reading, explaining that this involves believing you know what others think, and talk about how this might occur when you believe that others think you are weird or stupid.

To play the game, place all of the lotto cards on the table with the picture facing down. Explain how to play lotto if the child doesn't know. The rules are that you take it in turns to flip over a game card. If that card is on your board, you can place it on top of the matching picture on your board; if it isn't, you can turn it back over, leaving it where it is. You continue taking turns and filling your lotto board. The winner is the person to fill their lotto board first.

As you turn cards over, talk about the thinking error depicted on the card and provide an example of this that is relevant to the child. At the end of the session the child can take the lotto game home.

## What families can do

Helping parents to understand anxious patterns of thinking is important. It enables them to gently challenge their child's thoughts in the moment and also provides greater awareness of their child's experience. Parents can play a game as part of the session if they would like to do so. Alternatively, children can explain the game and talk with them about thinking errors toward the end of the session.

## Developmental considerations

This activity is most suited to older children who have a greater awareness of their thoughts and a better ability to challenge these.

# Thought error lotto template

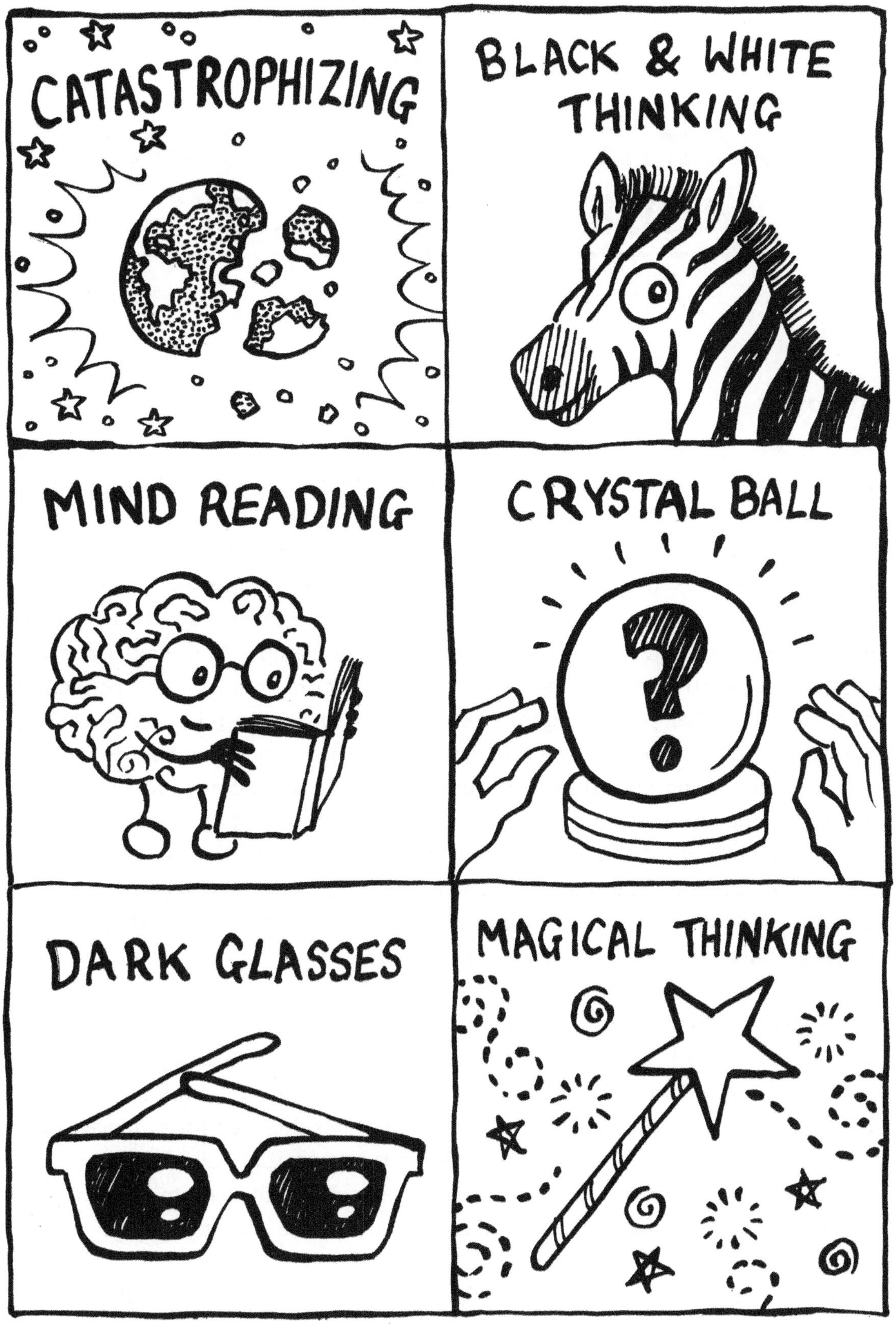

CATASTROPHIZING

BLACK & WHITE THINKING

MIND READING

CRYSTAL BALL

DARK GLASSES

MAGICAL THINKING

# CHAPTER 8

# FACING YOUR FEARS AND ACCEPTING ANXIETY

## AVERY

Avery (5 years) presented with a pattern of avoiding new activities. She had a black-and-white thinking style and was uncomfortable making mistakes. As a result, she avoided tasks she perceived as too difficult, including learning to ride a bike. Through therapy, Avery and her family were able to better understand her anxiety and appreciate how mistakes help us learn. During the sessions Avery had an opportunity to try a range of new activities through play, noticing her anxiety as she did so. Play also provided Avery with a space to begin gradually engaging in those activities she was worried about. For example, Avery engaged in doll play in sessions, helping the dolls to ride a toy bike for the first time. Sometimes the therapist chose to enact a character, pretending they were nervous about riding the bike and asking Avery what they should do or if she could say anything to them that might help. Her parents were encouraged to support her to play with her bike at home, purchasing a basket for it, which she enjoyed taking toys in and out of. On one occasion the therapist asked if Avery could bring a photo of her bike and new basket to the next session. Through play, Avery became gradually more comfortable and was then able to begin the process of slowly beginning to try her bike out at home. More generally, her parents and preschool teacher noted that her willingness to engage in other new activities had also increased.

The idea of being worried and doing it anyway is described throughout this book. This involves sitting with the uncomfortable feeling of worry while being able to understand it, know that it will pass and remember that sitting with this discomfort in the short term can be worthwhile in the longer term. It also implies the need for practice as it is often in that experience of being anxious and doing it anyway that a child begins to appreciate that they can do it and notices their worry dissipate. It is in that practice that they learn that doing what they are worried about can be worthwhile. Traditionally, practicing facing fearful situations is referred to as exposure.

Under a traditional cognitive behavioral approach, we tend to think about exposure as involving developing a hierarchy of fears and gradually facing the feared situations. This approach works particularly well with phobias in which it is easy to gradually work toward tolerating the feared stimulus. In our work with children, play often creates essential exposure, allowing the child to have a go and experiment in a developmentally appropriate way before facing the situation in their day-to-day lives. As in the example of Avery above, playing around a feared situation can create some anxiety in the clinic room and provides children with an opportunity to work through this and develop strategies for managing this more effectively. Indeed, play within the session provides a space in which children can gradually explore situations they find anxiety-provoking with a level of choice and control. Playing with a child in session also allows you to notice their feelings, helping them to name and regulate these in the room, as necessary.

Engaging in exposure tasks is difficult and therapists often describe sending children away to do this only to find that they have not done so. As with all the therapy we do, we need to be mindful that the child will be able to do more within the session than they can in their day-to-day life. The scaffolding and support we provide in sessions allows them to be able to do more than they can alone and the emotional intensity is likely to be less, meaning they can better access the thinking part of their brain. For this reason, engaging in some exposure through play in sessions is incredibly valuable. Once the child has had an experience of playing through a situation, they are often more likely to be able to engage in some exposure tasks at home. It is also important to remember that exposure needs to be supported by other techniques in therapy. When attempting exposure, we often help the child to use some calming strategies and may model some helpful thoughts. After the child has engaged in the activity they were worried about, we might help them evaluate the thoughts they had going into the situation, weaving in some cognitive work.

Some of the activities in this book are exposure-based tasks. For example, in *Scavenger hunt* (page 191), to assist with separation anxiety the child moves around the house and can gradually move farther away from the parents as we set increasingly distant items for them to collect. More generally most activities will elicit some emotions within the clinic room. For example, completing a craft activity for a child who is anxious can elicit a fear of making mistakes and a worry about it being perfect. Activities in which children talk about their worries often cause children to feel a little worried. Taking the time to notice and name these feelings of anxiety that arise, rather than being overly focussed on the content, is important. Helping a child to notice their body tensing and their voice rising, naming that as anxiety, and noticing that it lessens as the child continues with the task, is, at its core, exposure.

Trying to build a playful aspect into exposure tasks at home can also help. As with Avery, playful engagement with a feared situation often provides a safe first step. It takes the pressure off and reduces the child's and the family's anxiety. Explaining to parents the role of play in exposure is important as often they are overly focussed on the outcome, pushing the child too quickly to face their fears.

Often a traditional CBT approach involves developing a fear hierarchy in which steps are developed with the aim of helping the child to gradually face the situation they find anxiety-provoking. For example, a child who is worried about being away from a parent might begin with a step of playing in one room while their parent is in another for a few minutes. The way in which we develop fear hierarchies with children and families is included as an activity in our book *Creative Ways to Help Children Manage Big Feelings* (Zandt and Barrett 2017), and there are many other variations of fear hierarchies, stairways or stepladders in CBT-based anxiety programs (e.g., Bunge *et al.* 2017; Rapee *et al.* 2006; Stallard 2002). In practice, the act of developing a fear hierarchy can in itself be anxiety-provoking for children. Seeing all the steps laid out with the final endpoint being something that the child is fearful of and wants to avoid can reduce a child's likelihood of engaging with the steps. For these reasons, we often choose not to develop and outline a full fear hierarchy with the child and family, instead initially developing just the first step or two.

That said, there are some aspects of a fear hierarchy that are important for children and families to understand. First, it is important for children and families to know that we will be gradually working toward them doing those things that make them feel anxious. Second, it is important that the family understand that they will be involved in negotiating each step and that they choose something that is a good-sized step for them. Part of this is about creating an openness to sharing that sometimes the steps might feel too big or even too small, with the child and family being ready and willing to take on more. Each step can be negotiated flexibly. Third, it is essential that the child and family understand that they are likely to experience some anxiety with each new step, though that this will lessen over time. *Worry shrink ray* (page 193) is an activity that explores this idea.

This final point may seem obvious; however, for some families the idea of asking their child to do something that causes them anxiety seems counterintuitive and they will resist it. For example, some families have a belief that when their child feels relaxed they will be able to face challenges, and they believe that this is the first step rather than working gradually on the child facing their fears. Understanding a family's beliefs about anxiety and being able to articulate the notion that gradually facing fears helps to reduce the anxiety allows you to engage in some discussion around this before initiating the exposure process.

More generally, this allows us to have some discussion about whether or not we can protect our children from anxiety or whether what we want our children to understand is that you can be anxious and still do something; indeed, that doing something that makes you anxious can be worthwhile. We often tell children and families that everything worthwhile that we have done in our lives has caused us anxiety. Further, it provides a space in which we can talk about what it means to see yourself as someone who can face difficult and anxiety-provoking situations. It is often useful to help parents understand that when children do more, they feel more able to do more.

This is particularly true of a child's ability to manage new situations, tolerate change or handle uncertainty. Indeed, parents often try to minimize changes and create certainty for their children. While this is important, providing security and predictability, it does mean that when children are faced with a new situation they often have little experience of managing this. Although typically developing children generally manage changes well, children with anxiety can get caught up in their worry, finding the lack of certainty frightening. Indeed, intolerance of uncertainty is now a concept that we see being explored in research and related to anxiety in children (Osmanağaoğlu *et al.* 2018).

Children with autism spectrum disorders tend to have a particular focus on sameness, and recognizing this in their children, many parents go to added lengths to provide even greater certainty and predictability. Indeed, if it were possible to provide certainty and predictability for children for evermore, this might be the most advisable approach. In reality, however, children will be faced with changes and will have to tolerate uncertainty, and our ability to shield them from this will decrease as they move into the world of school and friendships. For example, children at school are frequently faced with changes of routine, and they often have to learn new concepts and must tolerate uncertainties, such as their classmates having a range of different opinions and there not being a single right answer. As such, a number of the activities in this chapter, including *Measuring change* (page 197) and *Unknown parcel* (page 199) focus on anxiety around changes and new situations, with a view to beginning to help children to tolerate and embrace uncertainty.

# Hurdles

Children who are anxious often avoid things they perceive to be difficult. This activity helps them think about facing challenges, using the metaphor of jumping hurdles.

## What you'll need

You will need some soft cushions that can be stacked (you will need to create some space for this in your clinic room, ensuring that the child is out of the way of any furniture or objects that they can bump into). You may also like to make a hurdle for the child to take home, using some popsicle sticks and glue.

## Introducing this activity

Wonder with the child about whether they have ever jumped hurdles and talk about what that was like. Explain that you sometimes feel like life is full of tricky things that can be a bit like hurdles. Suggest that you set up some hurdles together.

Demonstrate by talking about something that you find difficult and stacking the cushions up to make a hurdle. Talk with the child about how you might feel before jumping over this hurdle. For example, you might say, "I felt so nervous. My heart was pounding and my hands were shaking." You might also model some thoughts if this has been part of your work with the child. For example, "I thought I wouldn't be able to do it and then I remembered I could always try." Model that you can take a deep breath and try to jump the hurdle, reflecting on what it feels like when you have done so.

Encourage the child to think about something that is difficult for them and set up the hurdle so that they can have a go at jumping over it. Try to get the child to notice their feelings and thoughts prior to jumping, identify anything that will help them to get over the hurdle and reflect on how they feel afterwards.

If either you or the child is unable to jump the hurdle, this is a good opportunity to talk about how sometimes we need to jump a smaller hurdle first. You can then reduce the number of cushions and encourage the child to jump. Alternatively, you can talk about how we all need help sometimes and you can talk with the child about what would help them to jump the hurdle.

Some children will enjoy making a short video of themselves jumping over the hurdle, which can work well as a take-home option. Another option is to make a hurdle by gluing three popsicle sticks together as a reminder they can take home of the discussion you had. Children may like to use a marker to write something on the hurdle that they found useful in the discussion. This might be something like "Hurdles are part of life," "I'm good at jumping hurdles," or even "Breathe, then jump," depending on how they used the activity.

## What families can do

Parents of anxious children can feel reluctant about their child facing obstacles, so this is a useful activity for talking about what this is like for them. You can work up to talking about how obstacles are part of life and how we want our children to be able to have a go when faced with one.

Parents may like to identify an obstacle they have faced and have a go at jumping over it in the session, or they may like to watch their child doing so. Using this language at home (e.g., saying, "Oh that does seem like a bit of a hurdle doesn't it") is also a great way for parents to reinforce this idea.

## Developmental considerations

This is a great out-of-your-seat activity that appeals to both younger and older children. When completing this with younger children, you can choose a thought together that applies across different situations, such as "I can try," and have them say this out loud before they jump each hurdle. This modification often also works well with children with developmental difficulties. Similarly, the extent to which you talk about what you notice in your body and the complexity of the strategies you identify that can help with the hurdle will vary depending on the child's developmental level.

# Moldable brain

This activity helps children and families explore the concept of learning and mistakes, with a view to reducing the anxiety they may experience around this.

## What you'll need
You'll need some balloons in various colors and some soft modeling clay. You will also need a permanent marker or a pen.

## Introducing this activity
You can start this activity by noticing that the child's body or even their hair has been growing and ask about their brain and whether that has been growing too. Suggest that you make a brain together while you talk about how brains grow.

To begin making the brain, take one of the balloons and cut its neck off so that you can fill it with soft modeling clay. You will need to poke the soft modeling clay in with your finger or you can push it in with a pen. Notice how the soft modeling clay changes shape as you work with it, noting how flexible it is. When the balloon is reasonably full, take another balloon and cut the neck off before stretching it over the first balloon so that the opening with the soft modeling clay is covered and the first balloon is visible through the opening in the second balloon. Mold the balloon into a brain-like shape, leaving the space where the first balloon is visible at the bottom.

Show the child the brain and decorate it using a permanent marker or a pen. For example, you may like to draw a line down the middle to identify the two hemispheres, or draw some lines so that the top of the brain resembles the cerebral cortex.

Allow the child to have a play with the brain and encourage them to describe how it feels. When you have talked about how the brain feels bendy, flexible and moldable, explain to the child that this is how brains really are, noting that we are able to learn and grow throughout our lives. You might like to talk about some examples of ways in which your brain has grown of late and wonder about what the child has learnt lately. Talk about how one of the main ways in which our brain grows is through making mistakes and provide some examples of mistakes you have made and how they have helped your brain to grow. Help the child to think of some examples too.

You may like to encourage the child to squeeze the brain as a reminder of how their brain is growing when they are learning something new or when they are feeling anxious about making a mistake. Sometimes children will like to pair this with a helpful self-talk statement, such as "These mistakes are helping my brain to learn."

## What families can do
It's useful to explain this concept to parents and reflect on ways in which their brains are growing too. Helping parents to understand that mistakes help us learn is useful, and supporting them to think about what language they can use around mistakes at home is important.

*Your Fantastic Elastic Brain* by JoAnn Deak, illustrated by Sarah Ackerley (2010) is a great book that introduces children and families to the notion that their brains are constantly developing and learning. It pairs well with this activity and is a good option for something to send home with the family along with the brain you have made.

## Developmental considerations

Younger children may find it easier to squeeze their moldable brain when they are worried, using it much in the way you would a stress ball. Older children may enjoy learning more about the brain and could also use this brain model to talk about other parts of the brain, such as their feeling brain. The part underneath the brain where the first balloon is visible can be marked as the amygdala or feeling brain, depending on the language you have been using with the child.

# Hide and seek

Hide and seek is a universal game that is often played by children and parents. It involves a playful separation, which is typically followed by a joyful reunion. It is a wonderful game for children with separation anxiety as it allows them to practice separation in a safe context.

## What you'll need

You can play hide and seek within your clinic room; however, it is useful to be able to move beyond this if at all possible. For example, you might be able to extend the hiding space to the waiting room or the courtyard.

## Introducing this activity

Asking the family about whether they ever play hide and seek is often a good place to start. Once they have shared their experience with the game, you can suggest that you all play together.

Talk about who might hide and who will count first. If the child seems anxious, you may choose to have them hide with another person to start with. Talk about what it might be like to hide. What will it be like not being able to see Mom, for example? You can also talk about what it will be like to be looking for others and to not be sure where they are. Together, identify some of the things that might help when you are playing the game, such as taking a deep breath or remembering that everyone is safe.

Defining the hiding space is important. If you have any concerns about a child's ability to remain in the space, then limiting this game to your clinic room is important.

It is also important to be clear that if anyone wants to stop playing at any time then they can say, "Come out now" or similar, and everyone will come out of hiding.

When playing, try to tune into the child's feelings, naming their anxiety and modeling the strategies you have discussed. Some children may like to track their anxiety as they play and might, for example, be able to tell you afterwards that they felt less worried when they remembered that you were still in the building. When the child has the experience of finding their parent, you can reflect on those emotions too.

## What families can do

Ideally, parents will be engaged in the game of hide and seek, so the child can experience the playful separation from them as well as the reunion and reflect on the feelings that arise in both situations. Families can also play this game at home, and parents can be encouraged to tune into the child's feelings, naming them and modeling strategies for managing them.

## Developmental considerations

It is important to ensure a child's safety when playing this game. This is particularly important for younger children or those with developmental disabilities. Defining the hiding space and ensuring that children are not able to move outside this is essential.

# Scavenger hunt

Separation anxiety is often apparent in the home context, with children insisting on being within eyesight or staying in the same room as their parents. This activity helps children who have separation anxiety to feel more comfortable gradually moving away from their parents. It provides an opportunity to be away from their parents and feel ok about it because of the playful context. For children who feel anxious during the game, it provides an opportunity to explore the idea that they can still engage in activities that make them anxious and that doing so is often worthwhile.

## What you'll need
You'll need paper and a pen or markers.

## Introducing this activity
Say to the family that you've noticed that the child's worries about being away from their parents means that they are staying very close to them. Explain that sometimes playing a game can help with this and suggest that you make a scavenger hunt game together.

Ask if the child has ever done a scavenger hunt and explain what this involves. Talk with the child about how they will have a checklist of things to collect and it's a race to see who can collect them first. Suggest that you make two games—one to play in the session and one to take home.

Make a checklist together, initially of items that the child can collect in the room or elsewhere at the clinic. For a child who tends to remain on their parent's lap, collecting items from within the room is often sufficient. If the child is more comfortable in the clinic room, you might want them to collect items from the waiting room or garden, depending on the clinic set-up. For example, your checklist might include a pen, a doll from the dolls' house and a magazine from the waiting room. You can then make a number of copies of the list, one for each person who is going to play. Once the game starts, the aim is to be the first person to have collected all of the items on the list.

Try to notice the child's feelings as you talk about the game. Notice any changes of facial expression and body language and make guesses about how the child is feeling. If the child is reluctant to participate, talk about what might happen to their anxiety as they have a go. Suggest that winning the game might be worth being worried. You can also encourage them to choose the item on the list that they feel most willing to go and get and begin with that one.

When you are done, you can talk about how everyone felt. Talk with the child about whether they were worried and how this felt in their body. Ask about how those feelings changed as the game continued. For example, how worried did the child feel the first time they had a go at the game compared to the second? You can wonder too about whether it was useful to have something to keep them busy and whether having items to find gave them less time to focus on the worries. Asking about whether it was worth the worry is also often helpful.

You can then work together to create a checklist for a scavenger hunt at home. Try to include items that require the child to move around the house where they are likely to be away from their parents. For example, you could add a pillow from one of the bedrooms, something from their parents' room, or even a toothbrush from the upstairs bathroom.

Talk with the child about who is going to play the game and give the family enough copies to take home. It is also likely to be helpful to talk about when the family is going to play the game and review it next session.

## What families can do

This activity is best completed with parents in the room as they will be able to provide good knowledge of the family home and can help you to select appropriate items to find. Older children may be able to do likewise, though it may still be useful to run their lists past their parents prior to attempting the scavenger hunt.

This activity provides children with the opportunity to successfully move away from their parents for short periods of time. Parents can continue to build on this after the game. For example, encouraging a child to race to get something from their room while the parent times how long it takes is often something children who have played this game before will be open to.

More generally, it is important for parents to understand how their child staying close to them and avoiding any separation contributes to their anxiety, and how important it is to support their child to achieve small, manageable separations and gradually to build on these.

## Developmental considerations

Younger and older children tend to enjoy this activity. Older children will generally be more able to link the experience to their feelings of worry and to gain insight into the idea that it is often worthwhile and helpful to engage in activities that involve facing their fears. Younger children will need more parent support to make these links, and their parents' learning about their ability to manage separations and how they can support this moving forward is essential.

# Worry shrink ray

This activity helps children reflect on the importance of facing worries in small steps and encourages them to have a go at things even while feeling worried. This is particularly important for families who believe that the child will only be able to face feared situations once they are calmer. This activity can also help families understand the role of both avoidance and exposure in maintaining or overcoming anxiety.

## What you'll need

You will need scissors and either cardboard or craft foam to make into a shrink ray. You will also need markers, glitters and/or sequins for decorating it. You may like to use the *Shrink ray template* provided below.

## Introducing this activity

Talk about how you have noticed that sometimes the child has a really cool superpower and is able to shrink their worries. Notice, for example, that when they first came to therapy they seemed really worried and now they don't. Use your hands, holding them out to show how worried they were initially and then how worried they are now. Also let them know the changes you have observed in them. For example, you may notice that their shoulders now seem relaxed and that they are now happy to move away from their parents.

Express interest in this shrinking ability the child has and suggest that you make a shrink ray together. You can make a shrink ray by printing the template onto cardboard or you can draw one freehand onto cardboard or a sheet of foam. Color it in or decorate it with glitter and sequins.

As you are making the shrink ray, talk with the child about the worries they have shrunk and what has helped them to do this. Often children will say that they don't know what helped and that they "just did it." You can then reflect on how just trying an activity decreases worry about the activity and how the child was able to be worried and still have a go. Some children may also say that it helped them to breathe or talk with someone about this, and they may like to add these things as buttons or switches on the shrink ray.

Once the child is clear about how they have managed to shrink worries in the past, you can talk about ways in which they might be able to do this going forward. For example, you could say, "What would happen if you took your shrink ray when you started at your new school next week?" or "What's your guess about what's going to happen to your worries about swimming lessons once they start on Monday?"

## What families can do

It is helpful for parents to reflect on the importance of their child facing their worries or feared situations in a gradual and supported way, and to think about how they can help their child to do this. Parents can easily be involved in this activity—encourage them to talk about times they have felt worried or scared and still had a go, and the impact of this on their worries. If parents are not involved in the session, showing them the shrink ray and explaining how the child can shrink worries is often helpful.

## Developmental considerations

This activity is suitable for both younger and older children. With younger children it will be important to keep the language simpler and use examples that they are able to relate well to. Showing with your hands how big the worry was and how it shrank is particularly helpful for this age group. With younger children we would tend to focus only on how having a go can shrink your worries, whereas older children may like to think about other strategies that help. For example, they might talk about ways they can look after themselves or helpful things they can remember when in feared situations.W

# Shrink ray template

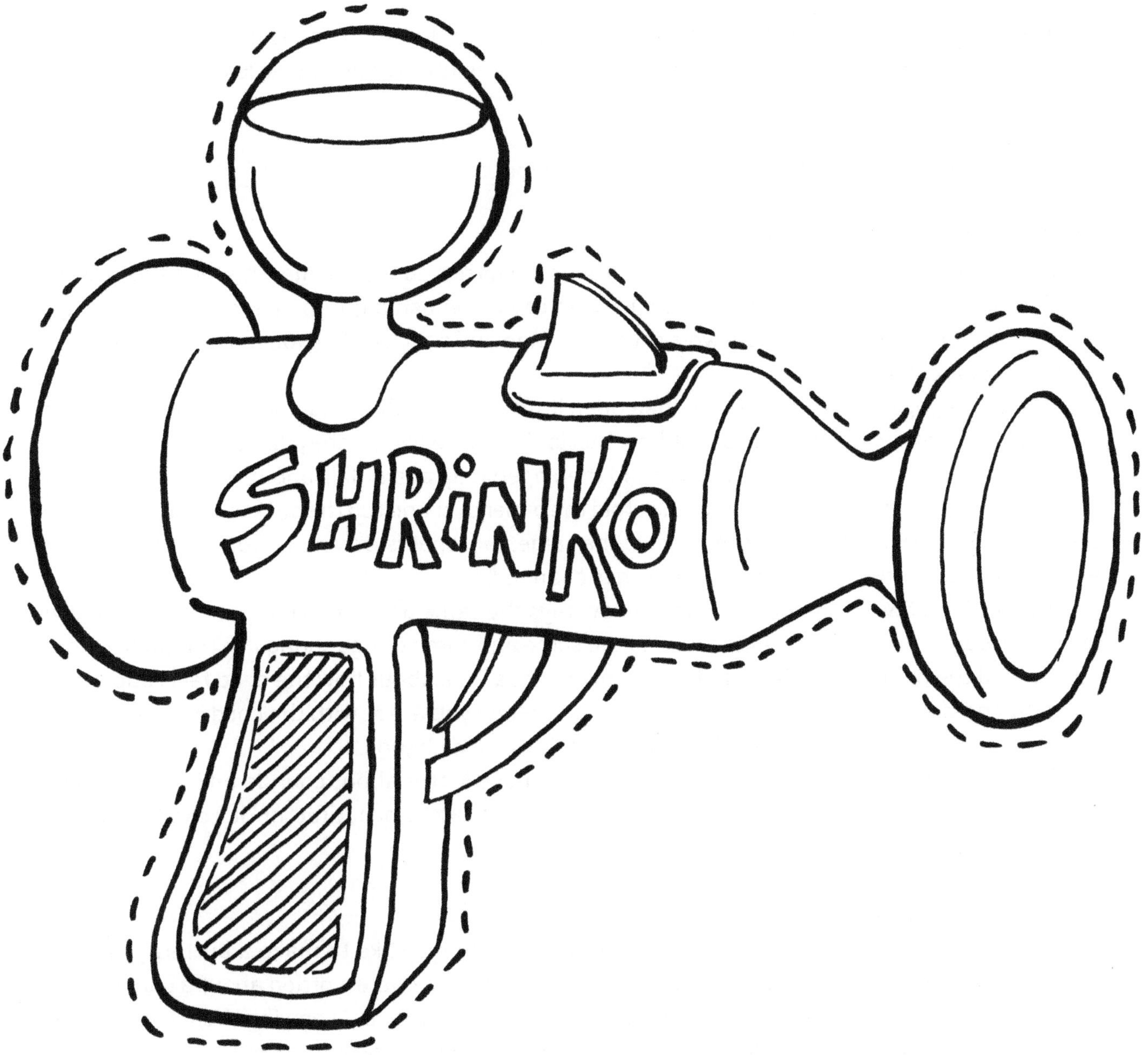

# Butterfly changes

Many anxious children worry about change and find it difficult to manage. This is a useful activity for helping children to think about change and manage the uncertainty it creates.

## What you'll need
You will need paper, and poster paint in a range of colors.

## Introducing this activity
Explain that you have noticed that sometimes the child worries about change. This might be related to starting in a new class, having a new child join their friendship group or even going through puberty. Explain that lots of people worry about change and suggest that you make some pictures to think about change.

Take some paper and fold it in half, then open it up and have the child dot some blobs of paint along one side of the crease. Talk about how this looks a little like a caterpillar and wonder about what will happen if you fold the page over and then open it up again. Talk about what might be the same and what might be different. Together, fold the paper over and rub the back of the paper before opening it up again. Notice together what is the same and what is different—for example, maybe all of the colors are still there but the shape has changed.

Repeat this a few times and talk about what stays the same and what changes. Reflect on how change usually involves some things staying the same and some things changing. The same colors remain and the paint is still there, but the form changes. Talk about how the child feels about the butterfly compared to the caterpillar. Depending on where you are at with the child in therapy, you can also talk about feelings in their body or thoughts around change.

Older children may like to write something they have learnt about change on the bottom of one of the pictures. This might be something like "Change can be beautiful" or "It's ok when things change."

## What families can do
Family members can easily be involved in this activity and may like to make a butterfly of their own. They might be able to share reflections of times when they were worried about a change and it worked out well. Talking with family members about the activity and showing them some of the paintings is another way to involve them in this. The paintings can be taken home and hung up as a reminder for children and families about these helpful messages about change.

## Developmental considerations
Both younger children and older children can engage in this activity. Younger children and those with developmental difficulties will need their parents to reinforce the ideas when they are faced with change at home.

# Measuring change

Children who are anxious often feel worried about new situations and can feel overwhelmed by change. This activity provides a space in which they can reflect on an upcoming change in a more balanced manner, contrasting what will change and what will stay the same. It is a helpful way to challenge a child's perception of a new situation and reassure them that they are able to cope with the change.

## What you'll need
You will need two long sheets of paper, Blu Tack® (poster putty) or tape to stick the paper to the wall, and markers or a pen.

## Introducing this activity
Say that you've noticed that the child is feeling anxious about an upcoming situation and reflect on how this is understandable given that there will be some change. Wonder about how much is going to change and how much is going to stay the same. Ask the child whether you could measure this together.

Stick the two sheets of paper to the wall, suggesting that you write all of the things that are changing on one piece and all of the things that are staying the same on the other. Children who are anxious are likely to focus more on what is changing, so list each of those things as the child names them. You might call this list "Changing." You can comment on how long the list is and empathize with the child for feeling worried about this. While you are talking, you might also like to talk about other aspects of worry, such as identifying what is occurring in their body or how big their worry is.

As you talk, begin to gently draw out things that won't be changing, adding these to the second list, which you might choose to call "Not changing" or "Staying the same." You may need to ask direct questions to elicit the items for this list and encourage the child to think more broadly.

For a child who is starting at a new school the lists may look like this:

# Changing

- new school
- new teachers
- new timetable
- new students.

# Staying the same

- my basketball team
- my family
- my friends in our court

- my house

- my computer club

- my dog.

Ask the child whether they can stand against the wall so that you can see how they measure up in terms of the changes. Even the longest of lists should be smaller than most children and this gives you an opportunity to comment on how the child is bigger than all of the changes and reflect some of their capacity and strengths. This is also a good opportunity to talk about some of the changes that the child has managed previously and reflect on how they have managed this.

## What families can do

Parents can feel similarly anxious about new situations, and many parents of anxious children worry about how their child will cope with change. This often adds to the child's sense that they will not be able to cope, so being able to look at this in a more logical manner together, and remembering that the changes are smaller than the child, helps parents and children alike.

## Developmental considerations

Younger children will enjoy this activity though they will need support to think about what is and isn't changing. For anxious younger children, completing this activity may be more therapeutic for their parents and should give their families a language to talk with them about change. Children with developmental difficulties are likely to need support to list specific aspects that are changing and those that aren't. Older children are also likely to enjoy this activity and will be more able to identify what is changing and what isn't.

# Unknown parcel

This activity helps children who feel anxious in new situations to have a more balanced perspective and promotes their ability to manage uncertainty. It also helps parents to understand that they don't need to provide excessive amounts of reassurance to their children when they are faced with new situations.

## What you'll need
You will need a small box or a paper bag to use for your parcel. You will also need paper and a pen. Something to decorate the parcel with can be fun, such as markers, ribbon or stickers.

## Introducing this activity
Explain to the child that you recently received a parcel in the mail and ask if they have ever had a parcel delivered to their house. Talk with them about what that was like—how did they feel when the parcel arrived, what about when they opened it? Ask if this was a parcel that they knew was coming or if it was a surprise. Ask about what it might be like to have a surprise parcel and not know what is inside. Talk about how most parcels have good things in them, though some are much more exciting than others. If we don't know what is in the parcel, we have no idea about what to expect.

You might use an example here from your own life. For example, I often talk about excitedly opening a parcel only to find that it was a replacement part for my food processor. On the one hand, I was disappointed that it wasn't something more exciting, like a surprise present; but on the other hand, I was pleased that I could now use my food processor again.

Talk with the child about how this is like new situations. Often we don't know what to expect. Sometimes new situations are wonderful, sometimes they are less enjoyable; however, they are usually ok. Make a parcel to serve as a reminder of this. You can make a simple parcel out of a brown paper bag or with a small box. Think about writing a message and putting it inside, such as "Even in new situations I am ok."

## What families can do
This activity also provides a way of talking with parents about how much scaffolding and support they might be providing for their child, and the value of children being able to manage uncertainty. You can talk with parents about how they can provide their child with the parcel without needing to describe what's inside. That is, they can provide a frame, such as "We are going to the beach on Saturday," but they don't need to provide details about exactly what will happen. For example, they might say, "If the waves are good, we might boogie board. Otherwise we might play in the rock pools." It is important to talk with parents about how important it is for their child to learn to manage some uncertainty and think about how the parents might be able to promote this.

## Developmental considerations
Younger children with reasonable language skills should be able to engage in this activity when supported to do so by their parents. Older children should easily be able to engage in this and tend to enjoy making a parcel.

Children with autism spectrum disorders find a lack of certainty particularly difficult, which can be challenging given that things change and life tends to be unpredictable. Working on this can be valuable; however, it is important that this is done in a supported manner. This activity can be useful as part of your broader work with these children.

# Box of chocolates

Many children struggle with uncertainty and find it hard to manage when things are not as they thought they were going to be. Some anxious children have a strong idea of how they want things to be and become anxious and angry when things are different. This activity helps children to think about uncertainty as part of life and to begin identifying ways in which they can manage when things happen in a way they weren't expecting. It uses the metaphor of life being like a box of chocolates—you don't know what you'll get. (Some families are familiar with this metaphor from the *Forrest Gump* movie.)

## What you'll need
You will need an empty chocolate box, cardboard in a range of colors (including brown), scissors, and markers or colored pencils.

## Introducing this activity
Talk with the child about your experience of eating a box of chocolates. The chocolates often come in different shapes and sizes. Some of them have delicious centers and some of them have strong-flavored or bitter centers. If you don't have a picture explaining which chocolates are which, you won't know what they are going to taste like. This means that you might end up with a chocolate that is different to what you thought.

Using an empty chocolate box, suggest that you and the child make some chocolates to go in the box. Make some chocolate shapes using cardboard and decorate them while you talk about what it's like to not know what something will be like. What is it like to bite into a chocolate and not know what the center will be? What is it like to try something new without knowing what it will be like? What sort of worries might that cause? What might that feel like in your body and what thoughts might go through your head? What can you do that helps?

Similarly, this activity is useful for exploring what happens when we expect something to be one way and it is actually another. For example, what happens if we think we are biting into a lovely strawberry cream only to find a hard hazelnut center?

Some children might like to write ideas about what helps in these situations on the back of their cardboard chocolates. Other children might like to make lift-the-flap cardboard chocolates, some of which have a nice surprise under the flap and others of which have centers that the child might not like. Others might like to write the quote from *Forrest Gump* on cardboard and paste it on the box as a reminder.

Making cardboard chocolates, like any craft activity, can elicit some challenges for children who are perfectionists, especially when the finished product doesn't look how they had wanted it to. Helping them to see the parallels between what they are experiencing and the activity itself is useful.

## What families can do
It is helpful for parents to understand that uncertainty is a part of life and the importance of building their child's capacity to manage it. Parents can join in the session, helping to make the chocolates

and reflecting on how they manage uncertainty and unexpected outcomes. At home, they can support their child by allowing them to face some uncertainty and assisting them to manage the anxiety it elicits, rather than seeking to avoid uncertain situations. Children can bring their box of chocolates home and show other family members, sharing the ideas.

## Developmental considerations

Younger children can engage in this activity, though they are likely to have difficulty linking the metaphor of the chocolates to uncertainty in their life. It may still be helpful to engage their family in the activity, to assist their parents to think about how uncertainty is part of life and how it impacts on their child, and to begin identifying ways in which they can support their child to manage when things happen in a way they weren't expecting. Older children can engage in more complex conversations about this concept and are likely to enjoy the activity.

As with the previous activity, this can be a useful way of helping children with autism spectrum disorders to manage uncertainty, though this needs to occur in a gradual and supported manner.

# Parting Words

Throughout this book we have presented a range of playful, practical and purposeful ideas for working with children with anxiety. We would encourage you to adapt the activities we've presented, modifying these so that they meet the needs of the children and families you work with. Reflecting on how the child and family experience the anxiety and how they learn best is also important when modifying activities.

Equally, it is important that you adapt the activities to suit your therapeutic orientation, the setting and context in which you work, and your individual therapeutic style. Surrounding yourself with colleagues who do similar work will allow you to learn from others and we strongly encourage supervision for all therapists, regardless of their level of experience.

Child and family work involves many challenges; however, it also has the potential to be incredibly powerful, with impacts that ripple well beyond the individual children you see.

Keep playing and learning!

*Fiona and Suzanne*

# References

Achenbach, T.M. and Rescorla, L.A. (2000) *Manual for the ASEBA Preschool Forms & Profiles.* Burlington, VT: University of Vermont Research Center for Children, Youth, and Families.

Achenbach, T.M. and Rescorla, L.A. (2001) Manual for the ASEBA School-Age Forms & Profiles. Burlington, VT: University of Vermont, Research Center for Children, Youth, and Families.

Adams, D., Clark, M. and Simpson, K. (2019) 'The relationship between child anxiety and the quality of life of children, and parents of children on the autism spectrum.' *Journal of Autism and Developmental Disorders.* Available at https://doi.org/10.1007/s10803-019-03932-2, accessed 01/31/20.

Ahlen, J. and Ghaderi, A. (2019) 'Dimension-specific symptom patterns in trajectories of broad anxiety: A longitudinal prospective study in school-aged children.' *Development and Psychopathology 32*, 1, 1–11.

Alderson-Day, B. and Fernyhough, C. (2015) 'Inner speech: Development, phenomenology, and neurobiology.' *Psychological Bulletin 141*, 5, 931–965.

Alfano, C.A. (2018) '(Re) conceptualizing sleep among children with anxiety disorders: Where to next?' *Clinical Child and Family Psychology Review 21*, 4, 482–499.

Alfano, C.A., Gonzalez, R. and Meers, J. (2019) 'Treatment of Comorbid Sleep Problems in Anxious Children.' In L. Farrell, T. Ollendick and P. Muris (eds.) *Innovations in CBT for Childhood Anxiety, OCD and PTSD: Improving Access and Outcomes.* Cambridge: Cambridge University Press.

American Psychiatric Association (2013) *Diagnostic and Statistical Manual of Mental Disorders* (5th ed.). Washington, DC: American Psychiatric Association.

Balcke, T. (2015) *I Have a Worry Colouring-In Book.* Richmond, NSW: Tanya Balcke.

Balcke, T. (2016) *I Have a Worry.* Richmond, NSW: Tanya Balcke.

Barrett, P.M. (1999) 'Interventions for child and youth anxiety disorders: Involving parents, teachers, and peers.' *Australian Educational and Developmental Psychologist 16*, 1, 5–24.

Beesdo-Baum, K. and Knappe, S. (2012) 'Developmental epidemiology of anxiety disorders.' *Child and Adolescent Psychiatric Clinics of North America 21*, 3, 457–478.

Benjamin, A.H. and Chapman, J. (2005) *Baa! Moo! What Will We Do?* London: Little Tiger Press. (Original work published 1996.)

Birmaher, B., Brent, D.A., Chiappetta, L., Bridge, J., Monga, S. and Baugher, M. (1999) 'Psychometric properties of the Screen for Child Anxiety Related Emotional Disorders (SCARED): A replication study.' *Journal of the American Academy of Child and Adolescent Psychiatry 38*, 10, 1230–1236.

Boer, F., Markus, M.T., Maingay, R., Lindhout, I.E., Borst, S.R. and Hoogendijk, T.H.G. (2002) 'Negative life events of anxiety disordered children: Bad fortune, vulnerability, or reporter bias?' *Child Psychiatry and Human Development 32*, 3, 189–199.

Bolton, D. (2005) 'Cognitive Behavior Therapy for Children and Adolescents: Some Theoretical and Developmental Issues.' In P.J. Graham (ed.) *Cognitive Behavior Therapy for Children and Adolescents* (2nd ed.). Cambridge: Cambridge University Press.

Bunge, E.L., Mandil, J., Consoli, A.J. and Gomar, M. (2017) *CBT Strategies for Anxious and Depressed Children and Adolescents: A Clinician's Toolkit.* New York, NY: The Guilford Press.

Carr, A. (2014) 'The evidence base for couple therapy, family therapy and systemic interventions for adult-focused problems.' *Journal of Family Therapy 36*, 2, 158–194.

Carr, A. (2016) *The Handbook of Child and Adolescent Clinical Psychology: A Contextual Approach* (3rd rev. ed.). London: Taylor & Francis. (Original work published 1999.)

Carr, A. (2019) 'Family therapy and systemic interventions for child-focused problems: The current evidence base.' *Journal of Family Therapy 41*, 2, 153–213.

Cattanach, A. (2008) *Narrative Approaches to Play with Children.* London: Jessica Kingsley Publishers.

Chorpita, B.F., Yim, L., Moffitt, C., Umemoto, L.A. and Francis, S.E. (2000) 'Assessment of symptoms of DSM-IV anxiety and depression in children: A Revised Child Anxiety and Depression Scale.' *Behavior Research and Therapy 38*, 8, 835–855.

Deak, J. and Ackerley, S. (Illustrator). (2010) *Your Fantastic Elastic Brain: Stretch It, Shape It.* Naperville, IL: Little Pickle Press.

De Los Reyes, A. and Makol, B.A. (2019) 'Evidence-Based Assessment.' In L. Farrell, T. Ollendick and P. Muris (eds.) *Innovations in CBT for Childhood Anxiety, OCD and PTSD: Improving Access and Outcomes.* Cambridge: Cambridge University Press.

Donovan, C.L. and Spence, S.H. (2000) 'Prevention of childhood anxiety disorders.' *Clinical Psychology Review 20*, 4, 509–531.

Driggs McLeod, A. (2018) 'Helping Sexually Abused Children Overcome Anxiety: A Play-Based Integrative Approach.' In A.A. Drewes and C.E. Schaefer (eds.) *Play-Based Interventions for Childhood Anxieties, Fears and Phobias.* New York, NY: The Guilford Press.

Ebesutani C., Bernstein A., Nakamura B.J., Chorpita B.F. and Weisz J.R. (2010) 'A psychometric analysis of the revised child anxiety and depression scale—parent version in a clinical sample.' *Journal Of Abnormal Child Psychology 38*, 2, 249–260.

Esbjørn, B., Bender, P., Reinholdt-Dunne, M., Munck, L. and Ollendick, T. (2012) 'The development of anxiety disorders: Considering the contributions of attachment and emotion regulation.' *Clinical Child and Family Psychology Review 15*, 2, 129–143.

Ewing, D.L., Monsen, J.J., Thompson, E.J., Cartwright-Hatton, S. and Field, A. (2015) 'A meta-analysis of transdiagnostic cognitive behavioral therapy in the treatment of child and young person anxiety disorders.' *Behavioral and Cognitive Psychotherapy 43*, 5, 562–577.

Farrell, L.J., Ollendick, T.H. and Muris, P. (2019) 'Preface.' In L. Farrell, T. Ollendick and P. Muris (eds.) *Innovations in CBT for Childhood Anxiety, OCD and PTSD: Improving Access and Outcomes.* Cambridge: Cambridge University Press.

Fliek, L., Roelofs, J., van Breukelen, G. and Muris, P. (2019) 'A longitudinal study on the relations among fear-enhancing parenting, cognitive biases, and anxiety symptoms in non-clinical children.' *Child Psychiatry and Human Development 50*, 631–646.

Fuggle, P., Dunsmuir, S. and Curry, V. (2013) *CBT with Children, Young People and Families.* London: Sage.

Ghandour, R.M., Sherman, L.J., Vladutiu, C.J., Lynch, S.E., Bitsko, R.H. and Blumberg, S.J. (2019) 'Prevalence and treatment of depression, anxiety, and conduct problems in US children.' *The Journal of Paediatrics* 206, 256–267.

Ginsburg, G.S., Riddle, M.A. and Davies, M. (2006) 'Somatic symptoms in children and adolescents with anxiety disorders.' *Journal of the American Academy of Child and Adolescent Psychiatry* 45, 10, 1179–1187.

Gray, P. (2011) 'The decline of play and the rise of psychopathology in children and adolescents.' *American Journal of Play* 3, 4, 443–463.

Hancock, K.M., Swain, J., Hainsworth, C.J., Dixon, A.L., Koo, S. and Munro, K. (2018) 'Acceptance and commitment therapy versus cognitive behavior therapy for children with anxiety: Outcomes of a randomized controlled trial.' *Journal of Clinical Child and Adolescent Psychology* 47, 2, 296–311.

Harros. R. (2019) *ACT Made Simple: An Easy-to-Read Primer on Acceptance and Commitment Therapy* (2nd ed.). Oakland, CA: New Harbinger Publications.

Hayes, L. and Ciarrochi, J. (2015) *The Thriving Adolescent: Using Acceptance and Commitment Therapy and Positive Psychology to Help Teens Manage Emotions, Achieve Goals, and Build Connection.* Oakland, CA: Context Press.

Hirshfeld-Becker, D.R., Micco, J.A., Mazursky, H., Bruett, L. and Henin, A. (2011) 'Applying cognitive behavior therapy for anxiety to the younger child.' *Child and Adolescent Clinics of North America* 20, 2, 349–368.

Hoffman, K., Cooper, G., Powell, B. and Benton, C.M. (2017) *Raising a Secure Child: How Circle of Security Parenting Can Help You Nurture Your Child's Attachment, Emotional Resilience, and Freedom to Explore.* New York, NY: Guilford Press.

Hoffman, K., Marvin, R., Cooper, G. and Powell, B. (2006) 'Changing toddlers' and preschoolers' attachment classifications: The circle of security intervention.' *Journal of Consulting and Clinical Psychology* 74, 6, 1017–1026.

Hollo, A., Wehby, J.H. and Oliver, R.M. (2014) 'Unidentified language deficits in children with emotional and behavioral disorders: A meta-analysis.' *Exceptional Children* 80, 2, 169–186.

Hudson, J.L., Anagnos, J. and Ingram, V. (2019) 'Evidence-Based Care of Anxiety Disorders in Children and Adolescents.' In L. Farrell, T. Ollendick and P. Muris (eds.) *Innovations in CBT for Childhood Anxiety, OCD and PTSD: Improving Access and Outcomes.* Cambridge: Cambridge University Press.

Huebner, D. and Matthews, B. (Illustrator) (2005) *What to Do When You Worry Too Much: A Kid's Guide to Overcoming Anxiety.* Washington, DC: Magination Press, APA.

Ironside, V. and Rodgers, F. (Illustrator) (2011) *The Huge Bag of Worries.* Sydney: Hodder Children's Books. (Original work published 1996.)

James, A.C., James, G., Cowdrey, F.A., Soler, A. and Choke, A. (2015) Cognitive behavioral therapy for anxiety disorders in children and adolescents. *Cochrane Systematic Review – Intervention.* Available at https://doi.org/10.1002/14651858.CD004690.pub4, accessed 01/31/20.

Johnstone, L. and Dallos, R. (2013) *Formulation in Psychology and Psychotherapy: Making Sense of People's Problems.* London: Routledge.

Kaslow, N.J., Broth, M., Smith, C.O. and Collins, M.H. (2012) 'Family-based interventions for child and adolescent disorders.' *Journal of Marital and Family Therapy* 38, 1, 82–100.

Kaufman, J., Birmaher, B., Brent, D. and Rao, U. (1997) 'Schedule for affective disorders and schizophrenia for school-age children – present and lifetime version (K-SADS-PL): Initial reliability and validity data.' *Journal of the American Academy of Child and Adolescent Psychiatry* 36, 980–988.

Kneer, K., Reinhard, J., Ziegler, C., Slyschak, A. *et al.* (2019) 'Serotonergic influence on depressive symptoms and trait anxiety is mediated by negative life events and frontal activation in children and adolescents.' *European Child and Adolescent Psychiatry.* Available at https://doi.org/10.1007/s00787-019-01389-3, accessed 01/31/20.

Knell, S.M. (2015) *Cognitive-Behavioral Play Therapy.* Lanham, MD: Rowman & Littlefield Publishers.

Kristensen, H., Oerbeck, B., Torgersen, H.S., Hjelde Hansen, B. and Brunn Wyller, V. (2014) 'Somatic symptoms in children with anxiety disorders: An exploratory cross-sectional study of the relationship between subjective and objective measures.' *European Child and Adolescent Psychiatry* 23, 795–803.

Lin, Y. and Bratton, S.C. (2015) 'A meta-analytic review of child-centered play therapy approaches.' *Journal of Counseling and Development* 93, 1, 45–58.

Lippert, M.W., Pflug, V., Lavallee, K. and Schneider, S. (2019) 'Enhanced Family Approaches for the Anxiety Disorders.' In L. Farrell, T. Ollendick and P. Muris (eds.) *Innovations in CBT for Childhood Anxiety, OCD and PTSD: Improving Access and Outcomes.* Cambridge: Cambridge University Press.

Livheim, F., Hayes, L., Ghaderi, A., Magnusdottir, T. *et al.* (2015) 'The effectiveness of acceptance and commitment therapy for adolescent mental health: Swedish and Australian pilot outcomes.' *Journal of Child and Family Studies* 24, 4, 1016–1030.

Macleod, E., Gross, J. and Hayne, H. (2013) 'The clinical and forensic value of information that children report while drawing.' *Applied Cognitive Psychology* 26, 564–573.

Manassis, K. (2016) *Cognitive Behavioral Therapy with Children. A Guide for the Community Practitioner* (2nd ed.). New York, NY: Routledge. (Original work published 2009.)

Manassis, K, Lee, T.C., Bennett, K., Zhao, X.Y. *et al.* (2014) 'Types of parental involvement in CBT with anxious youth: A preliminary meta-analysis.' *Journal of Consulting and Clinical Psychology* 82, 6, 1163–1172.

March, J.S. (2012) *Multidimensional Anxiety Scale for Children* (2nd ed.). Toronto, ON: MultiHealth Systems.

Maric, M., Willard, C., Wrzesien, M. and Bögels, S.M. (2019) 'Innovations in the Treatment of Childhood Anxiety Disorders. Mindfulness and Self-Compassion Approaches.' In L. Farrell, T. Ollendick and P. Muris (eds.) *Innovations in CBT for Childhood Anxiety, OCD and PTSD: Improving Access and Outcomes.* Cambridge: Cambridge University Press.

McEvoy, P.M., Nathan, P. and Norton, P.J. (2009) 'Efficacy of transdiagnostic treatments: A review of published outcome studies and future research directions.' *Journal of Cognitive Psychotherapy* 23, 1, 20–33.

Moroney, T. (2005) *When I'm Feeling Scared.* Fitzroy, VIC: The Five Mile Press.

Moroney, T. (2017) *When I'm Feeling Nervous.* Fitzroy, VIC: The Five Mile Press.

Nauta, M.H., Scholing, A., Rapee, R.M., Abbott, M., Spence, S.H. and Waters, A. (2004) 'A parent report measure of children's anxiety: Psychometric properties and comparison with child-report in a clinic and normal sample.' *Behavior Research and Therapy* 42, 7, 813–839.

Newby, J.M. and McKinnon, A.C. (2019) 'Transdiagnostic Approaches to the Treatment of Anxiety Disorders in Children and Adolescents.' In L. Farrell, T. Ollendick and P. Muris (eds.) *Innovations in CBT for Childhood Anxiety, OCD and PTSD: Improving Access and Outcomes.* Cambridge: Cambridge University Press.

Osmanağaoğlu, N., Cresswell, C. and Dodd, H.F. (2018) 'Intolerance of uncertainty, anxiety and worry in children and adolescents: A meta-analysis.' *Journal of Affective Disorders* 225, 80–90.

Pearcey, S., Alkozel, A. Chakrabarti, B., Dodd, H. *et al.* (2018) 'Do clinically anxious children cluster according to their expression of factors that maintain child anxiety?' *Journal of Affective Disorders* 229, 469–476.

Perry, B.D. and Dobson, C. (2010) 'The Role of Healthy Relational Interactions in Buffering the Impact of Childhood Trauma.' In E. Gil (ed.) *Working with Children to Heal Interpersonal Trauma: The Power of Play.* New York, NY: Guilford Press.

Perry, B.D. and Szalavitz, M. (2017) *The Boy Who Was Raised as a Dog and Other Stories from a Child Psychiatrist's Notebook: What Traumatized Children Can Teach Us about Loss, Love, and Healing* (2nd ed.). New York, NY: Basic Books. (Original work published 2006.)

Piaget, J. (2000) *Play, Dreams and Imitation in Childhood.* London: Routledge. (Original work published 1951.)

Polanczyk, G.V., Salum, G.A., Sugaya, L.A., Caye, A. and Rohde, L.A. (2015) 'Annual research review: A meta-analysis of worldwide prevalence of mental disorders in children and adolescents.' *Journal of Child Psychology and Psychiatry 56,* 3, 345–365.

Rapee, R.M. (2012) 'Anxiety disorders in children and adolescents: Nature, development, treatment and prevention.' In J.M. Rey (ed.) *IACAPAP e-Textbook of Child and Adolescent Mental Health.* Geneva: International Association for Child and Adolescent Psychiatry and Allied Professions.

Rapee, R., Lyneham, H., Schniering, C., Wuthrich, V. *et al.* (2006) Cool Kids Anxiety Program. Sydney, NSW: Centre for Emotional Health.

Rapee, R.M., Wignall, A., Hudson, J.L. and Schniering, C.A. (2000) *Treating Anxious Children and Adolescents: An Evidence-Based Approach.* Oakland, CA: New Harbinger Publications.

Rector, N.A., Katz, D.E., Quilty, L.C., Laposa, J.M., Collimore, K. and Kay, T. (2019) 'Reassurance seeking in the anxiety disorders and OCD: Construct validation, clinical correlates and CBT treatment response.' *Journal of Anxiety Disorders 67.* Available at https://doi.org/10.1016/j.janxdis.2019.102109, accessed 01/31/20.

Retzlaff, R., von Sydow, K., Beher, S., Haun, M.W. and Schweitzer, J. (2013) 'The efficacy of systemic therapy for internalizing and other disorders of childhood and adolescence: A systematic review of 38 randomized trials.' *Family Process 52,* 4, 619–652.

Reynolds, C. and Kamphaus, R.W. (2015) *Behavior Assessment System for Children, Third Edition (BASC-3): A Targeted Individual Assessment of Behavior and Emotions for Children and Adolescents.* Bloomington, IN: Pearson.

Siegel, D. and Bryson, T.P. (2012) *The Whole-Brain Child: 12 Revolutionary Strategies to Nurture Your Child's Development, Survive Everyday Parenting Struggles, and Help Your Family Thrive.* New York, NY: Delacorte Press.

Silverman, W.K. and Albano, A. (1996) *The Anxiety Disorders Interview Schedule for Children IV (Child and Parent Versions).* San Antonio, TX: Psychological Corporation/Graywind.

Spence, S.H. (1998) 'A measure of anxiety symptoms among children.' *Behavior Research and Therapy 36,* 5, 545–566.

Spence, S.H., Rapee, R., McDonald, C. and Ingram, M. (2001) 'The structure of anxiety symptoms among preschoolers.' *Behavior Research and Therapy 39,* 11, 1293–1316.

Spence, S.H., Zubrick, S.R. and Lawrence, D. (2018) 'A profile of social, separation and generalized anxiety disorders in an Australian nationally representative sample of children and adolescents: Prevalence, comorbidity and correlates.' *Australia and New Zealand Journal of Psychiatry 52,* 5, 446–460.

Stallard, P. (2002) *Think Good – Feel Good: A Cognitive-Behavioral Therapy Workbook for Children and Young People.* Chichester: Wiley.

Stallard, P. (2009) *Anxiety: Cognitive Behavior Therapy with Children and Young People.* New York, NY: Routledge.

Stuijfzand, S., Creswell, C., Field, A.P., Pearcey, S. and Dodd, H. (2017) 'Research review: Is anxiety associated with negative interpretations of ambiguity in children and adolescents? A systematic review and meta-analysis.' *Journal of Child Psychology and Psychiatry 59,* 11, 1127–1142.

Swain, J., Hancock, K.M., Dixon, A.L. and Bowman, J. (2015) 'Acceptance and Commitment Therapy for Children: A Systematic Review of Intervention Studies.' *Journal of Contextual Behavioral Science 4,* 2, 73–85.

Telman, L.G.E., van Steensel, F.J.A., Maric, M. and Bögels, S.M. (2018) 'What are the odds of anxiety disorders running in families? A family study of anxiety disorders in mothers, fathers, and siblings of children with anxiety disorders.' *European Child and Adolescent Psychiatry 27,* 5, 615–624.

Treisman, K. (2016) *Working with Relational and Developmental Trauma in Children and Adolescents.* New York, NY: Routledge.

Treisman, K. and Peacock, S. (Illustrator) (2019) *Binnie the Baboon Anxiety and Stress Activity Book: A Therapeutic Story with Creative and CBT Activities to Help Children Aged 5–10 Who Worry.* London: Jessica Kingsley Publishers.

Van der Giessen, D. and Bögels, S.M. (2018) 'Father–child and mother–child interactions with children with anxiety disorders: Emotional expressivity and flexibility of dyads.' *Journal Of Abnormal Child Psychology 46,* 2, 331–342.

van Niekerk, R.E., Klein, A.M., Allart-van Dam, E., Rinck, M. *et al.* (2018) 'Biases in interpretation as a vulnerability factor for children of parents with anxiety disorders.' *Journal of the American Academy for Child and Adolescent Psychiatry 57,* 7, 462–470.

Vygotsky, L.S. (1986) *Thought and Language.* Translated by A. Kozulin. Cambridge, MA: The Massachusetts Institute of Technology Press. (Original work published 1954.)

Wagner, A.P. and Jutton, P.A. (Illustrator) (2013) *Up and Down the Worry Hill: A Children's Book about Obsessive-Compulsive Disorder and its Treatment* (3rd ed.). Manchester, NH: Lighthouse Press, Inc. (Original work published 2000.)

Wauthia, E., Lefebvre, L., Huet, K, Blekic, W., El Bouragui, K. and Rossignol, M. (2019) 'Examining the hierarchical influences of the big-five dimensions and anxiety sensitivity on anxiety symptoms in children.' *Frontiers in Psychology.* Available at https://doi.org/10.3389/fpsyg.2019.01185, accessed 01/31/20.

Weems, C.F. and Costa, N.M. (2005) 'Developmental differences in the expression of childhood anxiety symptoms and fears.' *Journal of the American Academy of Child and Adolescent Psychiatry 44,* 7, 656–663.

Wei, C. and Kendall, P.C. (2014) 'Parental involvement: Contribution to childhood anxiety and its treatment.' *Clinical Child and Family Psychology Review 17,* 4, 319–339.

White, M. and Morgan, A. (2006) *Narrative Therapy with Children and Their Families.* Adelaide, SA: Dulwich Centre Publications.

Whitney, D.G., Shapiro, D.N., Warschausky, S.A., Hurvitz, E.A. and Peterson, M.D. (2019) 'The contribution of neurologic disorders to the national prevalence of depression and anxiety problems among children and adolescents.' *Annals of Epidemiology 29,* 81–84.

Wolff, F., Savitz, H.M. and Letourneau, M. (Illustrator) (2005) *Is a Worry Worrying You?* Terre Haute, IN: Tanglewood Press.

Woolford, J., Patterson, T., Macleod, E., Hobbs, L. and Hayne, H. (2015) 'Drawing helps children to talk about their presenting problems during a mental health assessment.' *Clinical Child Psychology and Psychiatry 20,* 1, 68–83.

World Health Organization (2019) *International Classification of Diseases for Mortality and Morbidity Statistics* (11th ed.). Geneva: World Health Organization.

Young, K. and Dovidonyte, N. (Illustrator) (2016) *Hey Warrior.* Australia: Hey Sigmund Publishing.

Young, K. and Dovidonyte, N. (Illustrator) (2018) *Hey Awesome.* Australia: Hey Sigmund Publishing.

Zandt, F. and Barrett, S. (2017) *Creative Ways to Help Children Manage Big Feelings: A Therapist's Guide to Working with Preschool and Primary Children.* London: Jessica Kingsley Publishers.

Zhou, X., Zhang, Y., Furukawa, T.A., Cuijpers, P. *et al.* (2019) 'Different types and acceptability of psychotherapies for acute anxiety disorders in children and adolescents: A network meta-analysis.' *Journal of the American Medical Association of Psychiatry 76,* 1, 41–50.